IN

D0648942

"OFFERS THE FACTS THAT CAN SAVE YOUR LIFE"

"**Matter-of-fact, and upbeat,** this book explodes the myth that death from cancer is inevitable.

"Giving **sound, solid information** about self-examination...is where this book excels...**different from the run-of-the-mill,** how-to-do-it anti-cancer book....Also gives information that you would ordinarily find only in a medical library. Potter describes the early warning signals.

"**Potter is an expert** who has assembled everything you need to know about cancer in a simple, easy-to-understand book."

— *The Washington Post*

How to Improve Your Odds Against Cancer

BY

John F. Potter, M.D.

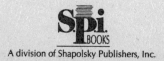

A division of Shapolsky Publishers, Inc.

S.P.I. BOOKS

A division of Shapolsky Publishers, Inc.

Copyright © 1992, 1988 by John F. Potter, M.D.

Previously published by Fell Publishers.

For any additional information, contact:

S.P.I. BOOKS/Shapolsky Publishers, Inc.
136 West 22nd Street
New York, NY 10011
212/633-2022 / FAX 212/633-2123

10 9 8 7 6 5 4 3 2 1

ISBN: 1-56131-076-8

Manufactured in the United States of America

~Dedication~

This book is lovingly dedicated to my wife Tanya and to our children; Tanya, Muffie and John.

～ Table of Contents ～

~Acknowledgments~

I am very grateful to Dr. Paul V. Woolley, III and to Dr. Edmund S. Petrilli for their reviews and comments on sections of this manuscript.

I also acknowledge the important contribution of Ms. Peggy McGovern, R.D., in compiling the diet schedules listed in the book.

Also, I extend my deep appreciation to Ms. Patrice Jones for her invaluable assistance in preparation of the manuscript.

John F. Potter

~Preface~

Cancer is afflicting and killing more Americans than ever before. This year, more than 960,000 people in this country developed cancer and 480,000 died from it. These are grim facts. But, the bitterest irony of this situation is that thousands of these victims should never have developed cancer, or they should have detected it at an early stage when the chance for a cure was good. To the physician, all deaths are distressing, but needless suffering and death are especially poignant.

As a surgical oncologist, I have seen the ravages which cancer can inflict. But, I can also tell you positively that you can decrease your chances of developing cancer by adopting a healthy pattern of living. Also, you can detect cancer early by performing self-examination of your skin, intra-oral tissues, breast, testes and other organs.

The first treatment of any cancer is all-important because it offers you the best chance that you will ever have for a cure. Consequently, it is critical that your first treatment should be based on the latest scientific knowledge and should be carried out aggressively. This book offers you advice on how to get such treatment.

Your psychological reactions on learning of a cancer diagnosis are essential to your well-being and are thoroughly discussed here.

The book follows the course of two hypothetical patients to illustrate these principles.

It is important that you know that not all cancers can be prevented or detected early, despite everyone's best efforts.

Nevertheless, you can—and should—take positive steps to improve your odds against cancer. This book tells you how to do this. Physicians avoid dramatic phraseology, but this information can be of life-or-death importance to you and to your family.

John F. Potter, M.D.

~ CASE STUDIES ~

Susan Webster was showering when she felt the lump in her breast. At first she thought—and hoped—she was mistaken. Again, she examined the area in the upper part of her left breast. This time, more slowly, she stroked the surface of the skin. Again, she felt a fullness, a thickening, a sense of resistance in this area. She experienced no pain or tenderness when she pressed on the lump, which was quite small, less than an inch in diameter. She repeated the examination several times.

Occasionally, she would feel nothing and was flooded by the hope she had been wrong; but after five minutes of gentle examination, she had come to the conclusion that there was something in her breast that had not been there before.

At the time, Susan was 36 years old and was an accountant

with a national accounting firm. She was single and had never been pregnant. She did not detect the lump in her breast by chance. Her mother had developed cancer of the breast in her mid-fifties and had eventually died of the disease. At that time, Susan's physician cautioned that she was at a slightly higher risk of developing breast cancer than the average woman because her mother had had this disease. He recommended she examine her breasts every month and suggested a yearly breast examination by a physician.

Susan had learned eight years ago, somewhat to her surprise, that she herself had fibrocystic disease. This benign condition is characterized by soft nodular thickenings in the breasts. As the months and years went by, however, Susan became quite familiar with these nodules, and they caused her little concern. Aside from a minor degree of discomfort just prior to her period, the condition caused her no difficulty. So, it was with some surprise—and even with a certain amount of clinical detachment—that Susan noted this new finding in her breast.

This detachment soon ebbed, however, and Susan's anxiety grew as she was driving to work. A feeling of disbelief replaced her clinical, cool assessment of the situation. She could not believe that this was happening to her. She reassured herself that this was probably nothing serious and that thousands of women had lumps in the breast and that the great majority of them were benign. Since her mother's illness she had read a great deal on the subject of breast cancer and she knew that this was indeed true—the odds *were* in her favor.

By the time Susan got to work, she was thinking clearly again; she wasted no time in making an appointment with her physician, the same internist who had cared for her for several years. At an office visit that very afternoon, the doctor examined her breasts carefully. He thought he detected a small tumor in her breast which seemed different from the fibrocystic nodules. However, he admitted he was unsure about this and he wanted Susan evaluated by a surgeon.

The following morning, Susan was seen by a surgeon. He believed that a tumor was present in the breast, and that the most prudent course of action was to remove it. He scheduled Susan for a biopsy which was to be performed under general anesthesia on an outpatient-surgery basis. He ordered a blood count, urinanalysis, chest X-ray, and EKG test which would be necessary before Susan could be put to sleep. He also ordered mammograms of the breasts. These X-rays were taken, as he explained to Susan, not to determine whether or not the lesions should be biopsied, but to determine whether there were any other suspicious lesions in either breast. This study, he added, was of value as a preliminary evaluation of a woman who was at increased risk of developing breast cancer, as was Susan.

The blood and urine studies, the chest X-ray and the EKG revealed no abnormality. The mammogram revealed fibrocystic disease but the radiologist was unable to detect a lesion which resembled cancer.

Two days after the test, Susan reported to the admitting office of a nearby hospital at 7:00 a.m. She had fasted since the previous night. She was examined by a surgical resident and an anesthesiologist, and then was taken to the operating room where she was anesthetized. The surgeon made a small circumferential incision over the mass and excised it along with a surrounding small area of normal breast tissue. The tissue was sent to the pathologist for a frozen-section microscopic examination. A few minutes later the pathologist entered the operating room. The diagnosis was cancer of the breast.

The surgeon met with Susan after the operation to explain that a small cancer, less than an inch in size had been removed. He explained that there was no evidence of any spread and that recovery chances for a patient with a tumor of this size were quite good. Nevertheless, further treatment of the breast, either by surgery or irradiation was necessary. He explained these treatment options to Susan carefully. She chose to have a modified radical mastectomy performed. On a subsequent admission to the hospital, this operation—the removal of the breast and the lymph nodes under the armpit—was carried out. Twenty such nodes were identified and none of them contained metastatic cancer. As a result no additional or adjunctive treatment was considered desirable for Susan.

****

The pain which eventually drove Todd McCormick to his doctor had begun, as far as he could remember, about five or six

3

months previously. Initially, he had noticed a vague discomfort inside the mouth near the left lower jaw. For many weeks he paid little attention to it. The discomfort, however, persisted and, in fact, became more bothersome. Todd started to take some aspirin to relieve the pain which was particularly troublesome when he was swallowing. As the weeks and months passed, he found himself increasing his use of aspirin; eventually he began to take codeine tablets which had been left over from a son's skiing injury the previous winter. Finally, Todd found it necessary to employ aspirin, codeine, and a shot of scotch to be able to get to sleep at night.

These symptoms had been present for about four months when he noticed when lifting his chin while shaving, that there was a lump in his neck just below his jawbone. This was the last straw for his wife who had been urging him to see his doctor for a number of weeks. Now, she took matters into her own hands and scheduled him for an appointment with his physician—an appointment which he kept.

Todd was 58 years old and was employed as a sales representative for a large aircraft manufacturer. He had been a fighter pilot in World War II and had seen action in Europe. While in the service, he had begun to smoke and drink. After the war, Todd stayed in the military as a pilot. He retired as a Lieutenant Colonel after 20 years of service and had little difficulty in obtaining his current position with the aircraft manufacturer. Now, he was smoking about a pack and a half of filter-tipped cigarettes a day, and his alcohol consumption was appreciable. At his rather frequent business luncheons, he had one or two martinis. While driving home in the evening he was yearning for his before-dinner drinks. Early in his marriage, he had persuaded his wife to have a pitcher of martinis ready when he got home. In recent years, however, she had been urging him to cut down on his drinking, and she had stopped preparing the drinks. Still, he usually had two drinks before dinner and a glass of beer or wine with his evening meal. Rather frequently, he would have a nightcap before going to bed. He was never discernably drunk in any business or social setting, nor had he lost time from work because of drinking, though frequently he was late getting to the office in the morning and really wasn't productive for a few hours. He rarely had need to see a physician and he believed he was in fine health.

Todd's physician found a large tumor present on the left side of the tongue in the back of the mouth. The tumor measured approximately 2½ inches long and 1½ inches wide. The physician noted that it extended from the tongue to the tissues in the floor of the mouth and then invaded the lower jaw bone. The swelling which Todd had noted in the mirror while shaving was a 1½ inch lymph node which the doctor thought contained metastatic cancer.

A biopsy of the intraoral tissue revealed a squamous cell cancer. Todd was seen and evaluated by a surgeon specializing in head and neck cancer and by a radiation therapist. Both realized that the prognosis for a tumor of this size and extent was not good. After considerable discussion, all parties decided that a radical operation was necessary. Todd was advised of the nature and extent of his illness and he was informed candidly that the prognosis was not promising. Nevertheless, there was no evidence to indicate distinct spread of the tumor was present and cure was still possible.

During surgery the tissues in the left neck, including the major muscle, the internal jugular vein and the lymph nodes, were removed. A portion of the jaw bone, the tongue and the floor of the mouth involved by cancer were also excised. A tracheostomy was done to place a temporary hole in the windpipe for the immediate post-operative period.

Todd recovered from this extensive operation quite promptly. He was ambulatory the next day and was fed through a tube into his stomach. His convalescence was good and both feeding and breathing tubes were removed within several days.

However, the pathology report received a few days after the operation was disturbing. Cancer cells were present in the lymphatic vessels in the specimen. The large node which had been previously felt in the neck and four other nodes were involved by cancer. The capsule of the large lymph node had been invaded and destroyed by cancer cells.

The prognosis for Todd was poor. After deliberation, it was decided that he was at high risk for recurrent cancer and that adjunctive radiation therapy should be initiated as soon as his wounds healed. Todd completed his course of irradiation, which was relatively uneventful, although he was troubled by inflammation of the lining of his mouth. This reaction subsided soon, however. His taste had been impaired by his treatments but he was eating a soft diet without difficulty. His speech and swallowing were satisfactory. He returned to work. He felt all right.

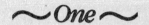

~ One ~

INTRODUCTION

There is a great chasm between the lives of those who have failed cancer treatment and those who have either never had the disease or who have been successfully treated. There are few instances in the human experience where the penalties which one group must pay are so severe in comparison with those of the other, more fortunate group.

Millions of Americans have failed cancer treatment. The price they pay is a high one. Deaths are usually slow and are accompanied by pain. Frequently this pain is excruciating and unrelenting. At the same time, the afflicted experience a gradual but inexorable loss of strength and body functions. Coupled with these physical penalties is the emotional distress their condition imparts—and this may be the harshest injury of all. They are aware of the disease and its outcome, and they suffer grievously from

7

this knowledge. Family and friends of the cancer victim share this oppressive psychological burden. A more mundane but still important consideration is the economic losses that cancer inflicts, especially when the patient is the breadwinner of the family. Ultimately, dying of cancer is a process which totally consumes both patient and family.

Those patients who do not develop cancer or experience it in their immediate families are in the minority in this country and they are fortunate indeed. Almost as well off are those who do develop cancer but overcome it with successful treatment. Millions of these Americans have been cured of cancer and now enjoy excellent health. Though they have paid relatively minor and temporary costs in pain and disability, these penalties have been exacted in the past and now they lead normal and productive lives.

Knowledge of the nature of cancer was, in the past, negligible. It was considered by some to be an inevitable component of the aging process. This led to the belief that cancer was caused by genetic factors inherent in the individual which would inevitably manifest themselves. This concept nurtured a feeling of fatalism about the disease; its cause was unknown and the selection of its victims was random and inscrutable. Nothing could be done to alter these fates.

Biomedical research of the last few decades has banished these myths. Although the precise causes and mechanisms by which cancer develops are not certain, our knowledge of cancer has increased impressively. Far from being helpless victims of an inexorable destiny, we know now that much of cancer is environmentally caused and, therefore, can be prevented.

If cancer does develop, its early detection is of critical importance in treatment. Early detection of a cancer greatly increases the prospects for cure and lessens the amount of suffering which cancer can inflict. The aggressiveness and length of treatment may be less for early tumors, and disability and loss of body function are also minimized by the detection of an early cancer. Finally, the economic costs for patient and family will be far less.

The stimulus to write this book has come from my all-too-frequent involvement with patients whose cancers were either preventable, or whose tumors could have been detected at a far earlier stage in their development. Certainly, it is a distressing experience to watch the suffering of a cancer patient who succumbs to the disease despite the best possible medical care; but, it is even more tragic to watch such a death when it should never have happened—when the cancer should never have developed, or when it should have been detected when cure was probable.

This book is designed for the layman. It will tell you what you can do to improve your chances against this disease, how to prevent cancer, and how to detect it early. It delineates what you can do to improve your own health.

Let me state promptly and clearly that there are types of cancer about which little can be done. We do not know how to prevent some forms of cancer. In certain organs, we are unable to detect cancer early in its development, despite our best efforts. It is not an uncommon experience to see a patient whose first symptoms occur when the disease is incurable.

Nevertheless, there is still great scope for improvement in cancer prevention and detection. This book focuses on those cancers which are common in occurrence, which are the major killers of our citizens, and against which effective action can be taken. It is estimated that prevention and detection efforts could influence the course of approximately 80 percent of the 900,000 people who will develop cancer this year in our country.

You probably are aware that an unprecedented commitment has been made by the American people, speaking through their Congress, to put an end to the suffering which cancer inflicts. The resulting support of basic and clinical research has offered new insights into the nature of this disease. These discoveries have, in turn, produced a steady improvement in cancer survival figures. At present, almost half of all patients who develop serious forms of cancer will be cured. This is an extremely impressive achievement. Nevertheless, prevention of the disease is our ideal goal and early detection will further improve current cure rates.

We Americans consider cancer to be our primary health problem. Certainly, there is much to fear from this disease. But, the irony of this situation is that knowledge is already available to dramatically improve the outlook in cancer, but too many people are not taking advantage of these opportunities. To avoid these mistakes, your keys to success are knowledge and the initiation of positive action. This book is written to allow you to tip the scales in your favor—to improve your odds against cancer.

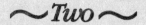

~ Two ~

The Magnitude of the Problem

In some way, cancer has probably affected every person in the United States. From personal experience you know that, all too often, cancer is afflicting members of your family, your friends, and members of their families. The magnitude of the cancer problem at the national level is no less disturbing.

The American Cancer Society has defined the scope of this situation. A sobering picture emerges from their findings:* ...

- About 74 million Americans now living—about 3 of every 10— will eventually develop an aggressive form of cancer.

Cancer Facts and Figures - 1987 published by the American Cancer Society.

- Three of every 4 families in this country will at some time know the emotional trauma of cancer.
- Currently, 5 million Americans have had—or now have—cancer.
- This year, about 971,000 people were diagnosed for the first time as having cancer.
- The statistics on deaths from cancer are equally disturbing. Approximately 483,000 Americans died of this disease this year, which means 1,323 people each day. One person succumbs to cancer every 65 seconds.
- The number of deaths from cancer is increasing steadily. In 1980, 414,000 people died of the disease. In 1981, the number was 422,000 and this figure has been rising steadily to the 483,000 deaths noted this year. By the year 2000 it is estimated that more than 500,000 deaths a year in this country alone will be caused by malignant tumors.
- There has been a steady rise in the age-adjusted national death rate. In 1930, the number of cancer deaths per 100,000 population was 143. In 1940, it was 152. By 1950, it has risen to 158 and in 1984, this number was 170. The major cause of these increases has been a devastating rise in the number of cases of lung cancer. This is particularly disturbing because this cancer is among the most preventable.
- Though cancer is claiming more victims, the cure rates for people who do develop cancer have been improving. For example, in the 1930s, fewer than 1 in 5 patients was cured of this disease. In the 1940s, it improved to 1 in 4 and by the 1960s the cure rate rose to 1 in 3. The most recent data indicates that almost half of all patients who get cancer will be alive five years after diagnosis. Obviously, however, there is still vast room for improvement with, at best, a 50-50 cure rate. About 170,000 people with cancer died this year who might have been saved by earlier diagnosis and prompt, effective treatment.

The cancer incidence for blacks is higher than whites and blacks also have a higher death rate. The American Cancer Society indicates that the overall cancer incidence rate for blacks went up 27 percent while for whites it increased 12 percent. Cancer mortality has increased in both races but the rate for blacks is greater than whites. In the last 30 years, cancer death rates in whites have increased 10 percent while black rates jumped 50 percent. The rates were virtually the same 30 years ago. Blacks experienced higher increases in incidence and mortality rates than whites in cancer of the lung, colon-rectum, prostate and esophagus. Esophageal cancer has shown an alarming increase in incidence in the black population.

You may be surprised to learn that cancer develops frequently in children. An estimated 6,600 new cases of pediatric cancer were diagnosed in the United States this year. With 2,200 children dying from this condition, cancer is the chief cause of death by disease in children between the ages of 3 and 14 years. Only trauma kills more children than does cancer.

Certainly, these data on the incidence and death rates of cancer are alarming. Yet, rather than paralzying you with fear, these statistics should galvanize you into specific action—action that will improve your odds against cancer. You can do this. We will tell you how.

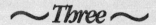

~ *Three* ~

The Biology of Cancer

Before you can improve your odds against cancer, it is necessary to know something about the nature of the foe. Cancer is a dangerous and implacable opponent, but you can often defeat it. As in any battle, it is extremely helpful to know your enemy. Knowledge about how cancer develops, how it grows and how it spreads will help you to prevent cancer and to understand its symptoms. Your ability to avoid cancer and to detect cancer early will be improved. Increasing your odds against developing cancer requires action on your part. Some of these actions are not easy and require a high level of motivation for success. Being aware of what cancer can and does do will help you in this effort. Knowledge of the biology of cancer forms the cornerstone of your intellectual and psychological commitment, and establishes a logical basis for your preventive actions. Psychological commitment motivates you to act on this knowledge.

Simply put, cancer is a disease of cell growth. To appreciate this phenomenon you must realize that the human body is composed of billions of cells. Each day sees the birth of millions of these cells. The cells grow to maturity and, after a period time, die. As cells die, or are damaged, they are replaced by new cells of the same type. Some type of innate control mechanism prevents excessive cellular proliferation and maintains equal balance between cell birth and cell death. The nature of this sophisticated control mechanism is essentially unknown.

In cancer, unfortunately, the control mechanisms either do not exist or have been overridden. Consequently, cancer cells multiply unchecked. The consequences of this wild proliferation—the spread of cancer—are all too well known.

We do not know what prompts this uncontrolled cellular growth or cancerous transformation. We do know, however, that a number of agents or factors are associated with it. Certain chemicals, for example, are known carcinogens, or cancer-producing agents. In the laboratory animal, cancer of the skin can be produced with regularity by painting the skin with coal-tar derivatives. X-ray irradiation has also caused cancer in certain situations. Viruses have been shown to cause cancer in laboratory animals and probably play a role in some types of human cancer. No matter which factor produces the cancer, the outcome is an alteration in the genetic information of the cell which causes it to undergo malignant transformation.

After a cell has become malignant, it begins to divide or proliferate unrestrainedly. Though the rate of growth of these cancer cells may not be unduly rapid, the process is inexorable. For a definite but unknown period of time, which probably varies for every tumor, the cancer will remain localized in the site in which it arises. During this important period, if detected and treated appropriately, the cancer would be completely curable. For example, it takes the average breast cancer cell several years to divide and grow to the size of one centimeter—which is less than half an inch. If the breast cancer could be detected at this early stage, it would be curable in the great majority of cases.

A cancer cell, however, has a number of characteristics which cause its lethalness. First, there is a decreased cohesiveness of one cancer cell to another. While normal body cells stick to one another rather tenaciously, changes in the membranes of the cancer cell impair such cohesion. This allows the cancer cell to detach itself readily from the host tumor and spread to other parts of the body.

Another dangerous characteristic of the cancer cell is its motility; it has the property of amoeboid motion, which is an undulating progress across tissue spaces that allows the cancer cell to invade adjacent tissue. These two characteristics—lack of cohesion and motility—are dangerous ones. They mean that cancer cells can separate themselves from their primary location and can infiltrate surrounding structures. This process of tumor spread—clinically defined as metastasis—has thus begun.

Conversely, a benign tumor does not have this capacity to detach itself and invade a neighboring tissue. The benign tumor grows until it encounters superior resistance and is then held in check. A malignant tumor, unfortunately, recognizes no such limitations and can, and will, and does, infiltrate relentlessly. This direct extension process is one of the characteristics that distinguishes the benign from the malignant tumor. In Todd McCormick, it permitted the cancer of his tongue to spread into the floor of the mouth and then into the jaw bone.

As the cancer enlarges, it may grow so rapidly that it outstrips its blood supply. Also, cancer cells may clog the vessels leading to the tumor. Consequently, the blood supply to the tumor becomes inadequate to sustain it and some cancer cells die. Unfortunately, this death of cancer cells occurs only in the center of the tumor; its periphery remains vital and continues to grow.

The cancer cell also has the capacity to invade the lymphatic vessels of the host organ. Once in these vessels, the cancer cells are then embolized or swept away in lymphatic fluid to adjacent lymph nodes. Here, they may grow to produce lymphatic metastasis. Spread of the tumor to a regional lymphatic node had occurred in Todd before he sought medical attention. This accounted for the tumor mass in his neck. This penetration of the lymphatic system is the second mechanism by which cancer spreads.

Additionally, cancer cells can invade small blood vessels around the tumor and thus gain access to the circulation of the body. Although their fates may vary, usually these cells are carried as emboli or tumor clots to a distant organ. Here, they become entrapped and arrested. Some of these cells may acquire a blood supply of their own in this new location and will continue to grow. Thus, a metastasis has been established by this process of hematogenous or blood-borne dissemination. This capacity of the cancer cell to detach itself from the primary tumor, enter the circulation and grow in a distant site, is its most lethal characteristic. Although not all cancer cells are successful in establishing themselves in their new environment, an all-too-high percentage of them do.

A final mechanism by which cancer spreads is known clinically as transcoelomic migration. This means that the cancer cells gain access to a body cavity, such as the peritoneal cavity in the abdomen or the pleural space around the lung, and drop off to establish distant spread. The classic example of this process, the so-called Krukenberg tumor, arises in the stomach and drops through the peritoneal cavity to implant in the pelvis.

One of the most important responsibilities of the oncologist—the physician specializing in cancer—is to determine the extent of the cancer's spread in the patient. This determination is known as staging, and is an essential feature in deciding the best form of treatment for the patient. Staging is a complex process and differs with each organ system. Nevertheless, generalizations can be made about the various categories of staging.

In broad terms, Stage I disease means that the cancer is confined to the organ of origin. There is no evidence of lymphatic involvement or vascular spread. This cancer is an early one and surgery or irradiation therapy would have a high probability of success. Although not all patients with apparent Stage I disease are cured, the cure rate is usually better than 80 percent. Susan's cancer of the breast would be categorized as Stage I disease.

Stage II disease is slightly more advanced. There may be evidence of spread to the regional or local lymph nodes adjacent to the tumor or evidence of greater growth in the primary organ. Nevertheless, this tumor is still regionally confined and offers a good prospect of cure with approximately a 50 percent five-year survival rate.

As the tumor progresses, however, it enters Stage III. Now,

there is a large and extensive primary cancer which has spread to adjacent structures, or there is evidence of extensive involvement of the lymph nodes. These lymph nodes may be fixed to one another or to surrounding structures. Surgery to treat this stage of cancer can be undertaken, but it is unlikely to remove all the cancer. Stage III disease offers a chance of survival by aggressive treatment, but the odds are not good. Five-year survivals run about 20 percent. This was the stage of Todd's disease when he was first seen by his physician. There was a large cancer in the tongue, which had fixed itself to the surrounding structures such as the jaw, and the tumor had embolized to establish a metastasis in the regional lymph nodes.

When there is evidence of spread to a distant organ, the clinician will define the lesion as Stage IV. In this situation, there is little chance for prolonged survival with most cancers and less than 10 percent of patients will be alive at the end of five years.

There are other clinical terms with which you should be acquainted. Cancer is synonymous with malignant tumor. There are two main types of cancers. Malignant tumors which arise from epithelial, or glandular, surfaces are called carcinomas. When a lining surface, such as is found in the skin or the inside of the mouth is involved, the cancer is called a squamous cell carcinoma. Glandular epithelium, such as that lining the colon or the stomach, creates a cancer called an adenocarcinoma.

When a cancer arises in connective tissue, such as bone, cartilege or fibrous tissue, it is termed a sarcoma. Such tumors are know respectively as osteosarcoma, chondrosarcoma and fibrosarcoma.

The pathologist is often able to analyze the microscopic appearance of the cancer cells and determine how mature or differentiated they are. The more mature the cell, the slower growing the cancer and the better the outlook for the patient. In general terms, a poorly-differentiated or undifferentiated cellular pattern suggests a rapidly growing tumor and a poor prognosis.

Cancer diagnosis is established on the histologic or microscopic appearance of the tumor. Tissue is obtained for this examination by a biopsy, which may be either excisional or incisional. In an excisional biopsy, the entire tumor, usually relatively small, is removed. When tumors are large and a diagnosis must be made before treatment can be planned, the surgeon may remove only a small portion of the tumor for study. This is called an incisional biopsy.

Another technique which is becoming of increasing value in cancer diagnosis is that of cytologic examination. Cytology is the study of the appearance of individual cells. A trained cytologist can determine by the appearance of the cell whether it is benign or malignant. The science of cytology was begun by Dr. George Papanicolau, who demonstrated the effectiveness of examining cells in the vagina for detection of cancer of the uterus. In the years since this monumental discovery, cytology has established itself as a superlative means for the detection of cancer of the cervix, enabling detection of these malignant cells before the cancer has begun to invade.

Untreated cancer, or cancer which doesn't respond to treatment, will ultimately produce death, though the exact mechanisms of death differ. The tumor may grow to prevent a vital function in the body, such as a cancer of the colon which causes intestinal obstruction. Other cancers may cause death by blood loss. Bleeding from a cancer of the stomach may cause the demise of the patient. When patients are unable to maintain proper nutrition in the presence of far-advanced cancer, their general body resources will be depleted and they may die of this effect. Finally, advanced cancer is associated with suppression of the body's immune system. This, and the general debility of the patient, predispose him to infection which may be the eventual cause of death.

Yes, this has been a grim recital of the stark reality about cancer. But you must remember it is possible in many circumstances to detect the cancer at an early stage of development before it has spread to distant sites in the body, and when, by effective treatment, a cure may be achieved. This is the objective of all physicians who treat cancer patients, and it must also be the goal of all of us who are vulnerable to this disease.

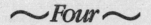

～*Four*～

An Ounce of Prevention ...

About 40 years ago, cancer was viewed as a disease linked primarily to the aging process and which was genetically determined. Since then, epidemiologic and other research studies have proven this belief inaccurate. In fact, a high percentage—some say up to 90 percent—of all cancers are associated with our environment. This means that the substances we inhale, the food and drink that we ingest, our exposure to radiation of a variety of types, and a host of other factors contribute to the development of cancer.

Perhaps the claims of environmentalists are excessive but it is certainly clear that a large proportion of our cancers are caused by the world in which we live and the way in which we live in it. While it is dismaying to learn that our environment is so noxious, this same realization has its encouraging aspects because it implicitly holds that elimination of these cancer-producing or carcinogenic factors will eliminate or decrease the development of malignant tumors. And, the prevention of cancer is vastly preferable to improvements in its treatment.

The prevention of cancer should be the concern, if not the preoccupation, of all thinking individuals. To help in that task, we will set forth the hazards in our environment which are currently known to be cancer-producing. You will learn how to diminish your odds of getting cancer by changing your patterns of living. You must be aware of the carcinogenic influences in your environment and how to avoid them if you are to improve your chances of avoiding cancer.

Certainly, the environment is not responsible for all cancer. Clearly, it is not. Each individual has an intrinsic resistance to cancer and that factor plays an important role in determining whether or not you will get this disease. Though you can do nothing to change your inherent susceptibility or resistance to cancer, you can do much to lessen your environmental risks.

~Five~

Tobacco

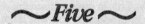

Tobacco was being cultivated by the Indians of North and South America when Columbus discovered the new world. Indians used tobacco in much the same manner as it is used today. But Indians believed that tobacco possessed medicinal value as did the Europeans who adopted this habit. Now almost 300 years later, we have established that, far from being medicinal in nature, tobacco is devastatingly injurious to our health.

Cigarette smoking has been unequivocally established to be associated with lung cancer. 150,000 cases of lung cancer developed in the United States this year alone. There were 136,000 deaths in this country this same year from cancer of the lung.

Until recently, lung cancer had been predominantly a male disease. Now, however, the marked increase in smoking among women since World War II has prompted a dramatic increase in lung cancer in females. The rise in lung cancer in women has occurred so rapidly that it is the most common cause of death from cancer in women.

Cigarette smoking is responsible for 85 percent of lung cancers in men and 75 percent of lung cancers in women. Those who smoke more than two packs of cigarettes a day have lung cancer mortality rates 15-25 times greater than non-smokers, according to a recent report by the Surgeon General. Lung cancer rates soar even higher for smokers who have been exposed to asbestos. Workers exposed to asbestos in the shipyard industry in the Eastern United States during World War II have had shockingly high levels of lung cancer. This combination of asbestos exposure and cigarette smoking increases an individual's lung cancer risk nearly 60 times.

Epidemiologists have also firmly established the frequency with which one smokes and the intensity and the depth of inhalation are major factors that increase the risk of developing cancer of the lung. Encouragingly, with the cessation of smoking, a gradual decrease in the risk of lung cancer ensues. After about 10-15 years, the ex-smoker has about the same risk for lung cancer as a non-smoker.

In addition to lung cancer, smoking has also been implicated in cancers of the mouth, pharynx, larynx, esophagus, pancreas and bladder. The American Cancer Society notes smoking accounts for about 30 percent of all cancer deaths, is a major cause of heart disease, and is linked to conditions ranging from colds and gastric ulcers to chronic bronchitis and emphysema. The Society also indicates smoking-related disorders are estimated to cause some 320,000 premature deaths each year. The Office of Technology Assessment of the U.S. Congress estimates the cost of smoking to the economy at $65 billion per year—about $2.17 in lost productivity and treatment costs for each pack of cigarettes sold.

Given all of this information, it is not surprising there has been a decline in the number of people who smoke. What is surprising is that, in light of all this, there are still so many who do. According to the National Center for Health Statistics, there was a decrease in smoking from 1976 to 1985, with the smoking rate among adult males over 20 years declining from 42 percent to 32 percent, and, among women, dropping from 32 percent to 28 percent. Still, the overall percentage of men and women in the United States who smoke is 30 percent. Each smoker smokes about 3,275 cigarettes per year down from 4,141. Nevertheless, in 1986, 584 billion cigarettes were smoked. Placed end to end, this number of cigarettes would encircle the earth approximately 1,500 times at the equator.

This unbelieveable consumption of cigarettes is mind-boggling, particularly when you realize lung cancer is extremely difficult to diagnose early and that, once the disease develops, it will kill about 90 percent of its victims within five years. Yet, people continue to die for a smoke!

Pipe and cigar smokers do not have the high-risks of developing lung cancer as does the cigarette smoker. The pipe and cigar individual has only a slightly higher risk of developing lung cancer than does the non-smoker. Presumably this is because people who smoke pipes and cigars do not inhale. However, before pipe and cigar smokers become too smug, they must be informed that their chances of developing intra-oral cancer—like Todd—are increased.

Much attention has been focused recently on passive smoking which occurs when individuals who live or work with people who smoke inhale the tobacco smoke produced by others. These passive smokers appear to have a slightly higher occurence rate of lung cancer than do individuals who do not live or work in such environments. This fact should—but in many cases doesn't—deter a member of the family from smoking, if only to protect his loved ones.

One unexpected, undesired and dangerous by-product of the campaign against cigarette smoking has been the increased utilization of chewing tobacco and snuff. Teenagers are taking to these habits with increasing frequency. Such use is no doubt prompted by advertising campaigns which feature sports heroes using chewing tobacco.

"Dipping snuff," as it is known, is a habit which is especially prevalent among women in the southeastern United States. In snuff-dipping, the user keeps finely ground or powdered tobacco tucked between gum and cheek. It is uncertain what factor in snuff causes cancer, but a prime suspect is N'-nitrosonornicotine or NNN,, which can produce tumors in laboratory animals. The NNN concentration in tobacco is raised even higher when the tobacco is mixed with saliva, presumably through the action of salivary nitrates. Snuff-dipping increases intraoral cancer rates 4 times and increases cancer of the gum and the buccal mucosa 50 times.

With the increasing popularity of smokeless tobacco, the output of this product in the United States has soared in recent years.

How to Stop Smoking

Articles, pamphlets, books and even videotapes have been produced about how to stop smoking. An extensive literature is available on such topics as the smoker's physical dependency on nicotine and the psychological addiction of smoking. Theorists have suggested the existence of different types of personalities, each of which has a different motivation for craving cigarettes. According to this approach, some smokers require smoking for stimulation, others for the sensorimotor manipulation of the cigarette-handling experience. Some have likened the depth of psychological grief experienced by an individual who quits smoking to the bereavement that accompanies the death of a family member or close friend.

To me, such studies attach far too much significance to the straightforward act of quitting smoking. If smokers needed any additional rationalization to avoid quitting—which they certainly do not—these concepts supply them with further excuses.

There have also been set forth lengthy lists of gambits which are intended to lessen the interest of the smoker in smoking and to ease the angst associated with quitting. These include such ploys as smoking only one-half of each cigartette, postponing lighting the first cigarette for one hour each day, buying cigarettes by the pack instead of the carton, and waiting until one pack is empty before buying another. Other suggestions include reaching for a glass of fruit juice instead of a cigarette and collecting all cigarette butts in a glass filled with water as a remembrance of your smoking past. Smoke ending clinics or programs can be of help. If these ploys work for you as an individual, please use any one or any combination of them.

There are some practical points to consider if you wish to stop smoking. First, it is very difficult to stop smoking if you are drinking. Also, with some people, smoking and drinking are so intertwined that alcohol use must be curtailed before smoking can be stopped. Also, it is difficult to stop smoking in a social setting where smoking is endemic. Stay away from friends who smoke while you are going through your transition period. Also, the effects of exercise are very beneficial and often compensate for the cessation of smoking. Finally, the effects of nicotine-containing chewing gum are said to be helpful, doubling the success rate of behavioral approaches, such as clinics.

The best reason to quit is because smoking cigarettes is monumental stupidity! Smoking destroys your health, decreases your enjoyment of life and robs you of years of life. Life is short enough and filled with enough illnesses without smoking. Deliberately adding to these burdens by smoking cigarettes is assinine. Studies designed to ascertain how one can motivate a person to stop smoking have not been very productive. What is needed in the anti-smoking campaign is to repeatedly remind smokers that they are impairing their health and to impress on them they have the free will to end this habit. There is much to be said for the benefits of self-discipline.

To put it succinctly: anyone who wants to stop smoking can. It is a matter of making up your mind to do so and then doing it. Amazingly, individuals who develop cancer give up tobacco with surprising ease; unfortunately, their decision is usually a little too late.

It isn't too late for you. Stop smoking now! At this moment. You can, if you want to.

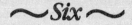

～ Six ～

Alcohol

The use of alcohol virtually dates back to the dawn of mankind. This drug, used in appropriate quantities and on suitable occasions, has helped man to cope with his condition and, in social and other settings, has enhanced his enjoyment of life. When abused, however, alcohol inflicts high penalities. The role which alcohol plays in the carnage on our highways is too well known to require comment. The alcoholic and his family suffer grievously in medical, social, psychological and economic realms. The relationship between excessive drinking and cirrhosis of the liver is common knowledge.

Not as well known, however, is the relationship between alcohol and the development of cancer. The cancers associated with alcohol abuse are those of the intraoral tissues, including the tongue, the floor of the mouth, the pharynx and the larynx. Also,

29

the frequency of cancer of the esophagus and of the liver is elevated in those who drink excessively.

The relationship between alcohol abuse and oral cancer is so striking that among doctors there is a flippant aphorism that if you encounter intraoral cancer in a person, the patient is probably an alcoholic. There are, of course, exceptions to this rule, but the generalization is reasonably valid. Studies performed on the epidemiology of oral cancer clearly implicate alcohol in the genesis of these tumors. However, since most heavy drinkers are also heavy smokers, it is difficult to distinguish precisely between the roles tobacco and alcohol play in the induction of these cancers. Rothman and Keller* meticulously studied 483 patients with cancer of the mouth and pharynx and compared them to 447 individuals without these cancers as controls. The authors calculated relative risks for different levels of alcohol and tobacco consumption and they discovered a marked increase in risk with the amount of alcohol consumed for each level of tobacco consumption and visa-versa. Alcohol and tobacco taken together in high quantities increase the risk of developing intraoral cancer 15 times in comparison to people who neither smoke nor drink. The precise mechanism by which alcohol and tobacco produce cancer of the intraoral tissues is unknown, but the fact that they increase your chance of developing these tumors is unassailable.

The converse of this situation is seen among groups such as Mormons and Seventh-Day Adventists, who either do not smoke or drink, or do so in a very limited fashion. The occurrence rate of intraoral cancers among these people is lower than in the at-large population, and is markedly lower than occurrence rates in people who smoke and drink heavily.

Todd is an unfortunate example of what can happen to an individual with heavy smoking and drinking habits. If Todd had kept his drinking within "reasonable" proportions and did not smoke at all, he probably would not have developed cancer of the tongue. Death from any form of cancer is usually unpleasant and often painful, but death from advancing cancer of the head and neck is particularly devastating. These patients suffer terribly not

---

Rothman, K. and Keller A. The Effect of Joint Exposure to Alcohol and Tobacco to the Risk of Cancer of the Mouth and Pharynx. J. Chronic Diseases 25:711, 1972.

only from the pain, but from physical disfigurement, difficulty in swallowing, speech impairment, bleeding, difficulty in breathing and drainage of pus and saliva. Intensifying this agonizing experience is that the patients are usually fully aware of their situation. The task of taking care of them in the hospital is difficult even for experienced health professionals; it is an overwhelming experience for family and loved ones to assist them at home.

Excessive use of alcohol is also well-established to be a causative factor in the development of cancer of the esophagus, particularly in black males. And alcoholic excess may lead to cirrhosis of the liver, which may lead to the development of cancer in this organ.

All of which, of course, leads us to a consideration of what is "reasonable" drinking. The extremes of the drinking situation, of course, are easy enough to define. The individual who has one or two drinks on a Saturday night needs to have little fear of the devastating effects of alcohol. At the other side of the spectrum is the person who would clearly be defined as an alcoholic by everyone—except possibly himself. This person is at increased risk.

It is consumption in the middle of the spectrum where the question of what level of drinking is harmful to your health becomes difficult to answer. To a certain extent, the answer would depend upon a number of factors including the type of alcohol consumed, how fast it is consumed, whether drinking was done with or without food, etc. There is also the important factor of individual resistance or susceptibility to the action of these carcinogens. There is great variation among individuals in regard to these factors. Unfortunately, the first indication that you will have that you are unusually susceptible to cancer is the development of a malignant tumor. At that time, this knowledge is of dubious value.

So, what is excessive drinking? To give you a definite answer, we consider more than two drinks daily injurious to your health. If you object to the stringency of these criteria, the question must be asked: "Why do you need more than two drinks a day?"

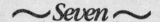

~Seven~

Diet and Nutrition

The role of diet and nutrition in the production of cancer has been a subject of increasing debate throughout the 20th century. Initially, there was considerable skepticism on the role foodstuffs played in the development of cancer, but in recent years thinking on this subject has changed. It is now considered quite likely that diet and nutrition do play a role in cancer induction. However, the problem remains that the evidence for this theory is not conclusive and it is difficult to determine precisely which dietary factors are significant. Nevertheless, the theory is too important to ignore; it may well be that simple modifications in your diet may improve your odds against developing cancer.

Three types of investigations are employed to study the relationship between diet and cancer: epidemiologic, which studies the occurrence of cancer in a human population in comparison to certain traits, such as diet; experimentation, in which modifications of diet are made in animals to see if the incidence of cancer is changed; and in-vitro tests, performed in test tubes to see if specific agents show cancer-producing properties.

Scientists study the results of all three of these methods in an attempt to further determine the relationship between diet and cancer. When the results of all three methods indicate the same conclusions, the determination is clear; however, when a discrepancy occurs between the results of these studies, it is difficult to draw a proper conclusion. For example, saccharin has been shown to be mildly cancer-producing in laboratory animals but has shown no such effect in epidemiologic studies in humans.

One problem with epidemiologic investigations of diet is that it is extremely difficult to know with great precision what people actually eat. Do you know exactly what you ate for lunch yesterday? Estimating the precise chemical composition of the allegedly eaten foods further complicates these investigations.

Despite all of these problems in methodology, however, a consensus on the relationship between diet and cancer is beginning to emerge. The first question that must be asked is whether the total amount of food eaten influences cancer induction. The evidence here is not clear. In the experimental animal, it does appear that animals with a reduced total food intake manifest a lower incidence of malignant tumors. The evidence in humans is less apparent, although in some studies there seems to be a direct relationship between obesity and increased occurrence of some cancers, such as cancer of the breast.

Other evidence suggests an increased amount of animal fat may be associated with increased occurrences of certain cancers, especially breast and large bowel. These conclusions were reached by analyzing the incidence and mortality rates from breast and colon cancer in populations with differing concentrations of dietary fat. For example, Japanese women have a low incidence of breast cancer in Japan, where the diet contains relatively little fat. When these women move to the West and adopt a Western diet with a high fat content, their incidence of breast cancer starts to climb. Laboratory research seems to confirm these observations. It has been shown in many animal tumor systems that increasing fat intake promotes the development of cancers in a number of organs.

It seems reasonable to speculate that Susan Webster's diet—high calorie, high fat, typical of affluent Western society—may have played a role in the development of her breast cancer.

Some evidence indicates that an increased protein intake may be associated with an increased risk of cancer. A substantial problem here, however, is that it is extremely difficult to differentiate the effects of high protein and high fat in the diet, as these two components are almost invariably linked. This means that the apparent association between a high protein load and cancer, may, in reality, be due to a high concomitant intake of fat, and not be protein-related.

The data on the relationship between carbohydrates or—starches—and cancer is too limited to draw any reasonable conclusions.

Recently, the importance of fiber, found in vegetables, fruits, and whole-grain cereals, has received great attention in both consumer and scientific publications. Studies have indicated high fiber diets are protective against the development of colorectal cancer.

The role vitamins play in cancer is a subject of incessant discussion in the media. There are protagonists of vitamins as preventative or curative measures for cancer; unfortunately, most of these pronouncements are not based on fact and are excessive in their promises of benefit. Nevertheless, evidence is beginning to accumulate that some vitamins may be of significance in the development or prevention of cancer. It appears that the incidence of cancer diminishes with an increase in the consumption of foods that contain Vitamin A, such as liver, or Vitamin A precursors, such as the carotenoids in dark green and yellow vegetables. These conclusions have been reached by the Committee on Diet, Nutrition and Cancer of the National Research Council.* The Commit-

Executive Summary: ..Diet, Nutrition and Cancer. Committee on Diet, Nutrition and Cancer. Assembly of Life Sciences, National Research Council, National Academy Press, Washington, DC, 1982.

tee, which carefully studied this area, concluded that Vitamin A itself, and many of the retinoids, are able to suppress chemically-induced tumors. It also found that foods rich in carotenes, or Vitamin A, are associated with a reduced risk of cancer. Be very aware, however, that Vitamin A is toxic in high doses and exceeding the levels of Vitamin A needed for optimum nutrition can be hazardous.

Studies have suggested that consumption of Vitamin C-containing foods, such as fresh citrus fruits and vegetables, may be associated with a lower risk of some tumors of the digestive system.

Clearly, there is no unequivocal evidence as to the role of diet in the causation of human cancer. Nevertheless, some investigators have estimated that diet is responsible for 30-40 percent of cancers in men and for 60 percent of cancers in women. Even if these scientists are only approximately right, diet is clearly a factor for consideration by the prudent person.

Consequently, it is important to follow some common-sense guidelines: . . .

Restrict total caloric and animal fat intake in your diet. Excess fat in the diet seems to be linked with increased occurrence rates of some cancers. Also, total caloric intake may have the same effect, independently. Restricting your diet as to both fat and total calories is a relatively easy thing to do.

Besides lowering your odds of developing cancer, caloric and fat restriction will also decrease obesity, which will facilitate diagnosis and treatment if any cancer does develop. A cancer measuring a half-inch in size is much more easily detected by patient or physician in a thin-breasted female than in a woman with large fatty breasts. Obesity plays a deleterious role in breast cancer detection. Also, obesity increases the difficulty of treating cancer, particularly for intra-abdominal cancer when treated by surgery. The surgeon has increased technical problems in operating on the obese patient. Operations which are simple in a slender individual may be more difficult in a person who is extensively overweight. The penalty for a patient's excessive weight may be longer time in the operating room, an increased occurrence of infection and other complications.

So, for a variety of reasons, cut down on your total caloric intake and the percentage of fat in your diet. These steps may well play an important role in preventing cancer, or in facilitating its treatment if it does develop. Additionally, these steps are also important as a general health measure because weight reduction and fat restriction will lessen your chances of developing cardio-vascular disease.

A second broad dietary guideline concerning prevention is that a high beta-carotene or Vitamin A intake is desirable. Foods rich in beta-carotene are carrots, deep yellow and green-leafy vegetables and yellow-hued fruit. Brussels sprouts and others of the cabbage family are believed to contain enzymes which inactivate or eliminate carcinogens, and these vegetables are therefore healthful; also whole grain cereals and fiber-containing substances are thought to decrease the occurrence of colon cancer.

Another important step is to minimize the consumption of salt-cured or smoked foods. There is epidemiological evidence that excessive consumption of smoked or salted products in countries such as Japan and Iceland is associated with markedly increased occurrence rates of cancer of the stomach. In fact, the occurrence of cancer of the stomach is very high in Japan, but declines in first-generation Japanese living in Hawaii. This strongly implicates an environmental and probably dietary factor in the induction of stomach cancer.

You can decrease your chances of developing certain kinds of cancers by adhering to fairly simple dietary guidelines. Control your body weight by restricting total caloric intake and the percentage of animal fat you consume daily. Increase your intake of dietary fiber. Eat more fresh fruits and vegetables. With such a balanced diet adopted, extensive supplementation of vitamins is not necessary.

Advice on Your Diet

Emphasize	*De-emphasize*
No excessive caloric intake— don't overeat	Excessive eating—keep calories in normal amounts
Fish, fowl, lean meat	High fat consumption both saturated and unsaturated

37

Diet and Nutrition

Emphasize	*Deemphasize*
Fiber in vegetables, fruits, whole grain cereals	Alcohol consumption
	Smoked foodstuffs
Vitamin "A" foods—liver, dark-green and deep yellow vegetables	Salt-cured or salt-pickled foodstuffs
Vitamin C containing foods—fresh citrus fruits and vegetables	Charred meat or fish
Cruciferous vegetables, e.g., cabbage, broccoli, cauliflower, Brussels sprouts	Charcoal broiling
	Nitrites and nitrates
Maintenance of normal body weight	

See the appendix for representative diets which incorporate these principles.

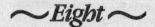

~ Eight ~

Sun

For more than a century, clinical evidence has abounded that excessive exposure to sunlight causes skin cancer. The high incidence of these cancers among sailors and farmers is evidence of this fact. Subsequently, it has been learned that the causative factor in skin cancer is the ultraviolet component of sunlight. Ultraviolet radiation, which is invisible to the naked eye, is that component of the electromagnetic spectrum which is shorter in wavelength than violet light. Of particular clinical concern is the so-called UV-B radiation which falls in the middle of the UV spectrum. A small quantity of this UV-B radiation escapes absorbtion by the atmosphere and reaches the earth's surface. UV-B produces sunburn in man and quickens the aging process of the skin in humans.

A thinning of the earth's ozone layer has occurred in recent

39

Sun

years. Ozone is one of the principal components of our atmosphere and protects us from excessive UV radiation by absorbing most ultraviolet light. Consequently, a decrease in the stratospheric ozone layer increases the amount of UV-B radiation reaching the earth. This so-called "ozone shield" is being depleted by the use of supersonic aircraft, nuclear weapons and nitrogen fertilizers. Halocarbons, commonly known as "freons", are inert gases used as aerosol propellants and as refrigerants which travel into the atmosphere and can destroy ozone. Depletion of the protective ozone layer must be regarded as a process that will increase the incidence of skin cancer.

Latitude or distance from the equator, also plays a very important role in the development of cancer of the skin. Direct measurement has established that there are marked increases in the amount of UV radiation by latitude. For example, in the winter, the UV count in Mauna Loa, Hawaii, which is located at 20 degrees north latitude, is 6,000. The count in Tallahassee, Florida at 30 degrees north is half of this, 3,000, and the counts fall progressively through other, more northern American cities. For instance, the UV count in Philadelphia, situated 40 degrees above the equator, is approximately 1,200, while the count in Bismarck, North Dakota, at 47 degrees is 1,000 (Scots, et al).

A study has shown there were far fewer skin cancers in Seattle, Washington, compared to 700 such cases in the Anglo population of Albuquerque, New Mexico. Another study demonstrates the incidence of skin cancer in Texas is 73 cases per 100,000 population, but only 58 in New York and 34 in Alaska.

Altitude is also a determining factor in the development of skin cancer. As the altitude increases, the atmosphere which acts as a filter decreases, and the exposure to ultraviolet light becomes greater. For each 1,000 meters increase in altitude, there is a 15 percent increase in ultraviolet rays that reach the surface of the earth. When low latitude and high altitude combine, as in Albuquerque, the population is subject to greater exposure to UV radiation and is more prone to skin cancer.

However, also of great importance is a person's inherent susceptibility or resistance to the effect of UV radiation. Skin cancer is a disease of whites, particularly of fair-skinned, blue-eyed blonds and redheads. Typically, these are the individuals who

40

sunburn while walking from the driveway to a beach cottage. They have great difficulty in developing a tan and their skin appears "thin." This blue-eyed blond or redheaded individual is frequently seen among Scottish and Irish populations and, therefore, these groups have a disproportionately high occurrence of skin cancer. An experiment in nature occurred when Great Britain established a colony in Australia. This social adventure exposed a population, ill-prepared by nature to meet it, to the implacable rays of UV radiation. As a result, the annual incidence of melanoma—a skin cancer—in Queensland, Australia is 14 males and 17 females per 100,000 population. This is an average annual rate of 16 melanoma per 100,000 population and is the highest reported incidence of this cancer in the world.

Conversely, the more darkly pigmented the skin, the greater the protection against the ultraviolet spectrum of the sun and the lesser the chance of developing skin cancer. Orientals, Latinos and particularly Blacks have very low incidences of these diseases. This diminished rate is believed to be related to the protective role of melanin, a pigment in the skin. The more melanin in the skin, the darker the skin is and the greater the protection against ultraviolet radiation.

Another contributing factor in skin cancer is the American lifestyle which has changed appreciably in the last 50 years. First of all, people have greater time for leisure activity, often in the sun. Clothing has become progressively more scanty and the parasol is a thing of the past. Furthermore, current mores apparently demand extended periods of sunbathing ... the current desideratum is a mahogany-colored hide.

It is no surprise, therefore, that the incidence of melanomas is rising very sharply in this country. An annual increase of about 8 percent is taking place. In just over a decade, the occurrence rate of melanoma has doubled. Disturbingly, melanoma in some patients may run a very aggressive course.

Simple common sense measures decrease your chances of developing skin cancer. Use these measures, especially if you are at increased risk for developing these tumors —if you are a blue-eyed blond or a redhead. Be cautious about excessive exposure to the sun. During the summer, you should, if possible, limit your exposure to the direct rays of the sun between the hours of 10 in

41

Sun

the morning and 2 in the afternoon. During this time, the sun's rays are directly overhead and the UV spectrum is filtered by only 15 miles of atmosphere. In the early morning and late afternoon, however, the sun's rays enter obliquely through the atmosphere and the depth of protective filtration is markedly increased.

Wear protective clothing, such as a hat with a broad brim for good protection of the head and neck area.

Use protective sun screens. There are a number of such preparations on the market and those with para-aminobenzoic acid (PABA) are particularly effective. The strengths of these sun-blocking agents have been graded as to their Solar Protection Factor (SPF). There numbers range from 2, the weakest, to 35, the strongest. Select the appropriate number for your individual needs. An SPF of 15 is very effective. They can be chosen to allow either gradual tanning or no tanning at all. The choice of the appropriate number should depend upon your individual suscep-tibility to the sun's rays.

Avoid sunburn at all costs. Not only is sunburn uncomfortable but there are some who believe that this sudden, intensive ex-posure to the sun may precipitate the development of a melanoma. This theory states that the more chronic or prolonged exposure to the sun such as that experienced by the farmer is more likely to produce basal cell or squamous cell cancers of the skin. These tumors, though not so worrisome as a melanoma, are cause for some concern, nevertheless.

Historically, we have considered melanoma as a disease of those age 40 and beyond. However, one clinician's experience indicates that younger and younger patients—some only in their early twenties—are being seen with melanoma. This would sug-gest that cautions against excessive sun exposure must be carried out with your children. Parents should instruct their young chil-dren to avoid sunburn. Adolescents should be made aware of the dangers of prolonged sun exposure. Make sure your children are aware of the importance of sun-blocking agents, especially at the beach. Behavior modification is much more easily made in child-hood; help your children to develop a prudent approach to the sun.

Again, the importance of common sense must be empha-

42

sized. There is no need for women to use a parasol and men a bathing suit extending down to above the knee. You can and should enjoy outdoor activity in the sun, but this should be done safely. Wear as much protective clothing as feasible. Don't lie around for endless hours in the sun. Even if baking in the sun does not result in skin cancer, your skin will age prematurely and you will look like a prune prior to age 50. Sit in the shade instead of in the sun. A simple measure such as wearing a polo shirt on the beach could be a life-saving measure for the individual at high risk because melanomas that arise on the trunk in males have a particularly aggressive growth potential, yet may be minimized by this simple step.

You can acquire an attractive tan but do it sensibly. Depending on your own complexion, begin slowly with 20 minutes of exposure on front and back on the first day. Gradually increase your period of exposure. Once you have acquired a tan that is good for you, avoid further sun-bathing. About all you will be achieving with excessive exposure is damage to your skin.

Another possible hazard in the development of skin cancer is utilization of suntanning lamps. The proponents of this approach suggest that the UV radiation which they employ is not carcinogenic. However, the use of this apparatus is of such short duration that its long-term effects cannot be safely predicted. Once more, caution is recommended.

With appropriate precautions you can enjoy the sun of summer as much as any one else while at the same time minimizing your risks of developing cancer of the skin.

~ Nine ~

Chemicals and Cancer

For more than 200 years, we have known that chemicals can cause cancer. In 1775, Sir Percival Pott, a London physician first noted the occurrence of the cancer of the scrotum in chimney sweeps of that city. This was the first demonstration of the carcinogenicity of coal-tar chemicals. The daily exposure of chimney sweeps to the coal-tar in soot, coupled with their economic and social status, which precluded adequate hygiene by a daily bath, led to chronic irritation of the skin by soot lodged in the folds of the scrotum.

These chimney sweeps paid a high price for the opportunity of gaining a livelihood. They developed cancers which led to their death simply because they were ignorant of the carcinogenic potential of coal-tar compounds in soot and because they didn't remove these carcinogens with a daily bath.

Although the public health problem of cancer in chimney sweeps has long since vanished, the dilemma of chemicals and cancer persists and has been magnified a thousand-fold. There are, at the present time, about 4 million known chemicals, both natural and synthetic; more than 60,000 chemicals are commonly used; and more than 1,000 new chemicals are introduced each year.

Some aspects of these statistics are indeed frightening. For example, the role of asbestos in cancer development has only been recently been recognized. Consequently, of the estimated 1 million current and former asbestos workers in this country, between 300,000 and 400,000—a startlingly high 30-40 percent—will die of cancer. The carcinogenic risk of asbestos is heightened by cigarette smoking; a long-time asbestos worker who also smokes cigarettes has a 60 times greater chance of developing cancer of the lung than does the average person.

Fortunately, as far as is known, the overwhelming majority of chemicals do not cause cancer. In fact, relatively few substances have been shown to produce malignant tumors. Most chemicals—even those which are demonstrated to be toxic or otherwise dangerous to your health—do not cause cancer. For example, in one study, 120 pesticides and industrial chemicals were tested at the highest possible doses in laboratory mice. These chemicals had been chosen because they were suspected of being carcinogens. Nevertheless, after two years of such testing, only 11 of these chemicals caused cancer in test animals.

Carcinogens are defined as cancer-causing agents, either synthetic or naturally occurring, which may be found anywhere in our environment. They may be concentrated in occupational situations where they are either used in the manufacturing process or are developed as a result of it. Almost invariably, cancer develops very slowly after exposure to a carcinogen. Cancers in humans usually appear 5 to 40 years after exposure to a cancer-causing agent. This long interval between the exposure and the development of a cancer is termed the latent period, and is one reason why it is difficult to incriminate a specific carcinogen with a particular cancer.

The manner in which chemicals induce cancer is quite complex, because the development of a tumor proceeds through the processes of initiation and promotion. A chemical initiator given to an animal does not, by itself, cause cancer, but does begin this process. Subsequently, a promoter, which may not, by itself, cause cancer, does induce malignant growth when given to the animal which has received the initiator. To compound the confusion, there may be individual factors of a genetic or viral nature also at work.

Clearly, the detection of carcinogens in our environment is a herculean task. This detection is accomplished by both in-vivo (involving living subjects) and in-vitro (test tube) studies. Among the in-vivo methods of detecting carcinogens are clinical observations by the physician, such as the observation by Pott of cancer in chimney sweeps. More sophisticated approaches are epidemiologic studies which seek to relate a significantly increased occurrence of a cancer to a specific agent. Also, there are experimental animal bio-assays in which a chemical suspected of being carcinogenic is given to a rat or mouse for a prolonged, usually life-time period. This method, although time-consuming and expensive, is one of the most valuable methods of determining carcinogenicity. Of all the known human carcinogens, all but two (benzene and arsenic) test positive as carcinogens in rodent bio-assay.

Although bio-assays have good scientific correlation with human cancer, the practical problems for evaluating chemicals by this method are substantial. The standard rodent assay of a single compound requires about 600 hundred animals studied over a two-year period, at a cost of more than $400,000. Also, assays often require a high dose of the agent and the data are obtained in only two specific strains of rat and mouse. Unfortunately, there can be significant differences in carcinogenicity between various strains and species in response to any specific theoretical carcinogen. Thus, the presence of a carcinogen might be missed by utilizing the wrong test system.

In an attempt to quicken the search for carcinogens and to decrease its expense, a number of in-vitro, or test-tube types of assays, have been developed. The most popular of these is the Ames Test, which exposes a suspected carcinogen to a culture of bacteria to see if a genetic change in the bacteria develops. If such a mutagenic change occurs, the chemical is considered a potential carcinogen and is subject to further, more extensive testing. The

47

Ames assay has shown to be correct in about 90 percent of cases in which it was used for both carcinogens and non-carcinogens.

A number of chemicals are associated with the development of cancer in man. Exposure to benzene increases the occurrence of leukemia; benzidine and Betanaphthylamine have been linked to the development of bladder cancer; vinylchloride has been shown to increase the occurrence rate of a rare tumor in the liver called an angiosarcoma; arsenic and coal-tar products have been shown to increase the incidence of skin cancer.

Some relatively simple steps will offer substantial protection against these and other chemicals. Most importantly you must be informed about the nature of the chemicals to which you are exposed. Are they carcinogenic and, if they are, what can you do to minimize exposure?

At work, follow the rules! Wear proper safety clothing and use appropriate safety equipment, such as a mask, if work regulations call for it.

Don't eat or drink in an area where chemicals are present. Don't get overconfident because you haven't gotten ill when you have violated safety instructions—remember that chemical carcinogenesis takes years to develop.

At home, know what chemicals are in your environment, and what they can do to you. Avoid long exposure to household solvent cleaners, cleaning fluids and paint thinners. Some of these may be hazardous if inhaled in high concentrations. Also, be careful and follow the instructions when using chemicals such as pesticides, fungicides and other garden and lawn chemicals. Keep these agents away from small children.

Keep the 200-year-old example of the chimney sweeps in mind—if appropriate action had been taken, these cancers could have been prevented.

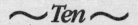

~ Ten ~

Venereally Associated Cancer

Cancer of the Uterine Cervix

Cancer of the cervix is a venereally-associated disease. This has been known for decades. The tumor's development is linked in some way with the act of intercourse. That knowledge allows us to take steps to lower the incidence of cancer of the cervix.

The cervix is the cylindrical neck of the uterus which projects downward into the vagina, and is covered by a thin layer of flattened cells called squamous cells. Carcinogenic influences can transform these normal cells into squamous cell cancer.

Through extensive epidemiologic investigation, we now know what factors and events cause marked increases in the risk of developing cancer of the cervix. One of the first observations was that cancer of the cervix was almost non-existent in virgins; in fact, the disease is extraordinarily rare among nuns.

From this observation, the relationship between intercourse and cancer of the cervix was analyzed. A key finding was that the age of the woman at the time of her first coitus correlated very closely with risk of developing this cancer. Women who became sexually active before age 20 have a two- to three-fold increase in the risk of developing cervical cancer in comparison to women whose initial sexual experience occurs later. The earlier the first act of intercourse, the greater the risk of this cancer. Why is this so? The adolescent cervix appears to be more susceptible to the action of carcinogens than is the cervix of the more mature female.

The number of sexual partners a woman has is also strongly related to an increased risk. This type of information is analyzed epidemiologically by studying women with multiple marriages, separations and divorces. Women with multiple marriages or partners have a two- or three-fold increase in the risk of developing cancer of the cervix in comparison to women with only one partner. Cancer of the cervix is common among prostitutes.

Whether or not the woman's partner is circumcized is also a factor in the induction of cervical cancer. The low incidence of cervical cancer observed in Jewish women prompted this speculation. Data suggests there *may* be a slighly lower incidence of this cancer among the partners of circumcized males. Lack of circumcision, therefore, is considered to be only a slight risk factor for the development of cervical cancer, and is more a matter of penile hygiene than circumcision.

Importantly, these studies focus upon the role of the male in the induction of cervical cancer and attempt to determine the precise mechanism of this process. Although the possibilities include the action of a chemical carcinogen in smegma, the role of viral infections venereally transmitted seems more likely.

It is more difficult, however, to make any strong assertions about the relationship between contraception and cervical cancer because so many variables and confounding factors are present. Users of oral contraceptives may have a higher prevalence of cervical cancer than users of the diaphgram. Clearly, the sexual practices of the woman will affect factors other than the choice of the method of contraception, making it very difficult to attribute an increased incidence of cervical cancer to type of contraception alone. Generally, there may be a slightly increased occurrence rate of cancer of the cervix among the users of oral contraceptives than among users of barrier methods.

The possibility that cancer of the cervix is caused by an infectious agent has received extensive study in both clinical and laboratory settings. A number of viral agents have been identified as links in a not-yet-fully defined manner in the development of cervical cancer. Human papilloma virus (HPV) has also been identified in a high percentage of cases of cancer of the cervix. The genetic footprint of this virus has been seen not only in cancer cells in the cervix, but also in lymph node metastases from such cancers. HPV has also been identified in benign neoplastic changes in the cervix which frequently progress to cervical cancer.

Herpes simplex virus 2 (HSV-2) has also been found in these cancers and this virus may act as a co-factor in producing the disease.

The implication of these studies is that a viral agent is transmitted during intercourse, causing cellular changes in the cervix which, in certain woman, progress to cancer.

Cancer of the cervix is a socio economically linked disease, whose frequency is much higher in women of lower socieconomic groups. Though the disease has been found in high incidence in the black population in this country, this association is due primarily to socieconomic status rather than to race, since the occurrence rate in poor whites is similar.

The incidence rate of cancer of the cervix differs widely in various countries in the world. In the United States, it has become relatively uncommon, almost certainly due to the benefits of Papanicolou screening (more commonly known as the Pap Smear) which permits early detection of neoplastic changes in the cervix and allows prompt treatment. The opposite situation is found in countries such as in Latin America where the disease is endemic and is the leading cause of cancer-related deaths among women. Latin American women have a three- or four-fold higher occurrence rate than white women in this country.

The conclusions from these observations is straightforward. Although the precise mechanisms of tumor transmission and induction have not been fully established, cancer of the cervix is certainly a venereally-associated disease. With the changing social mores in this country, increasing numbers of women are initiating sexual activity early in their lives; consequently, some of them will develop neoplastic changes in the cervix, which, as you remember, precede cervical cancer. The genital tract of the adolescent female may not have matured sufficiently to achieve an effective level of resistance to venereally-transmitted carcinogenic factors. Prudent personal and public policy would demand that this critical hazard of early initiation of intercourse be clearly delineated to these young women. Though such educational programs may be ineffective in delaying the onset of sexual activity, we are obligated to make this effort. A certain percentage of young women, so informed and counseled, will heed this advice.

Kaposi's Sarcoma

In the last few years, an extraordinary rise in the occurrence of a previously rare skin cancer—Kaposi's sarcoma—has developed in the United States. This rise has been caused by striking occurrence patterns in patients with AIDS (acquired immune deficiency syndrome). Kaposi's sarcoma results from an impaired immunological resistance in these patients.

Until recently, Kaposi's sarcoma was very rare in this country and was only infrequently fatal. Previously, the disease typically occurred in elderly men in their 60s and 70s. The disease, which ran a very slow and chronic course, was characterized by the appearance of purplish spots on the arms and legs. Only very rarely did the tumor invade or metastasize to distant organs, and most cases of this unusual tumor were observed in elderly men of Ashkenazi Jewish or Italian origin.

However, the type of Kaposi's sarcoma that has recently burst upon the American scene is dramatically different. It appears in patients with AIDS and runs an alarmingly and lethally different course. This disease is very aggressive, and can and does cause death by its rapid metastases to distant organs.

Other cancers of uncommon incidence are also being seen

in the AIDS population. These include Burkitt's lymphoma, squamous cell cancer of the tongue and cloacogenic carcinoma of the rectum. These tumors have been noted among male homosexuals in the past but their incidence appears to be increasing during the current AIDS epidemic.

From the point of view of cancer prevention, the implications for promiscuous homosexual males and for intravenous drug abusers, who also develop AIDS, are obvious.

~ Eleven ~

X-Ray and Cancer

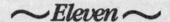

X-ray irradiation—from both natural and man-made sources—is a well-recognized carcinogen.

Natural sources of radiation include cosmic rays from the sun, which vary by altitude, and terrestrial radiation which varies geographically according to the natural occurrence of isotopes such as uranium in the earth. This natural, or background, irradiation can be responsible for the induction of human cancer, as evidenced by the Schneeburg mineworkers who developed an exceptionally high occurrence of lung cancer from unwitting exposure to uranium.

Radon is a colorless, odorless, radioactive gas which seeps from natural uranium deposits in the earth. Inhalation of radon can cause lung cancer. Previously, the radon problem was thought to be confined to small areas in the western United States. For example, homes in Grand Junction, Colorado and Butte, Montana, were found to have unsafe levels of this gas. But recent reports indicate radon is much more widely distributed than had been suspected.

High levels of radon have been detected in the "Reading Prong" area of western Pennsylvania and parts of New Jersey and New York. In one Pennsylvania housing subdivision, radon levels were 675 times higher than allowed by federal safety guidelines. Clearly, this is a dangerous situation. All in all, 30 states are encountering radon problems. It must be emphasized that this radon is emanating from naturally-occurring sources of uranium in the earth; it is not coming from radioactive waste dumps which are a well-recognized and well-documented concern.

The single most important man-made radiation factor is medical X-ray. Nuclear power and fall-out from nuclear weapons testing make only a minor contribution to the overall impact of man-made radiation. Radiation is responsible for only a very small part of the total number of cancers which develop in this country. Before the hazards of radiation were realized, X-rays were commonly used to treat non-cancerous diseases. For example, more than 30 years ago, approximately 14,000 patients were treated in British radiotherapy clinics for a benign rheumatoid condition of the spine known as ankylosing spondylitis. Subsequently, the death rates for these patients showed a significantly higher-than-expected occurrence of leukemia and excessive cancer rates were noted in other heavily-irradiated organs—particularly the lungs and pharynx—about ten years after exposure.

Increased rates have also been observed in women given radiation therapy for post-partum mastitis, an infection of the breast which develops after after giving birth. Breast cancer subsequently developed in these women at a rate twice that of a comparison group.

Similarly, radiation therapy used for the treatment of such childhood conditions as enlargement of the thymus gland, ringworm of the scalp, enlarged tonsils and acne resulted in an increased incidence of thyroid cancer which developed 5-35 years after exposure.

Obviously, then, therapeutic irradiation—the use of high-dosage X-ray for treatment purposes—can play a role in the development of subsequent cancer. Though body organs differ in their sensitivity to X-ray, all types of cancer appear to increase after irradiation, except chronic lymphocytic leukemia and possibly Hodgkin's disease and cervical cancer. Particularly, breast, thyroid and bone marrow appear to be the most sensitive areas, and the most likely to develop subsequent cancer.

Fortunately, the dosage of diagnostic X-ray—such as that used by physicians and dentists—is far less than that employed for treatment purposes.

Still, you should avoid undue X-ray exposure and have X-rays taken only for substantial reasons. Though physicians order X-rays only after due circumspection and on appropriate indications, it is certainly your perogative to query the reason for ordering a diagnostic X-ray. As regards dental X-rays, current thinking suggests that the frequency of routine X-rays should be based on the presence or absence of dental disease. If caries or periodontal disease is present, X-rays on a yearly or every-other-year basis would seem appropriate. In the absence of such disease states, routine X-rays should be obtained probably about every 5 years. Remember that although X-ray irradiation is a carcinogenic agent, in usual medical and dental circumstances it is not a significant cause of cancer.

In the future, other modalities of diagnostic imaging, such as ultrasound and nuclear magnetic resonance, will decrease the need for X-ray examinations.

Be aware of the possibility that the area in which you live may have high levels of natural radiation. An inquiry to your local, state or federal environmental protection office should furnish useful information on this matter. These offices will also have advice on what can be done to improve the safety of your home if elevated levels of radioactivity are present.

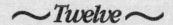

~ Twelve ~

Drugs and Cancer

Drugs are chemicals used in the treatment of disease. In the overwhelming majority of cases, these drugs promote your health and have led to increased lifespans. Nevertheless, drugs are chemicals which can have adverse reactions. One of these adverse effects is the induction of cancer, and a number of drugs have been implicated as carcinogens.

Estrogen

Estrogen, the female sex hormone, has been known to produce cancer in the laboratory animal for many years. Since estrogen preparations have been used for prolonged periods of time by millions of healthy women—sometimes in high dosage levels—it is important to understand the relationship of this hormone to cancer.

Drugs and Cancer

Between four and six million American women have been exposed to diethylstilbesterol (DES), a synthetic estrogen hormone, during pregnancies. First prescribed about forty years ago, DES was used in the first trimester of pregnancy—and frequently in high dosages—to treat complications of pregnancy including vaginal bleeding with risk of possible miscarriage, maternal diabetes and other less well defined situations. It was not until the mid-1950s that the results of a controlled clinical trial cast doubt on the efficacy of DES in managing these pregnancy complications, and the use of the drug began to decrease.

In 1971, an unusually high incidence of a rare type of vaginal cancer was reported in the daughters of women who had been treated with DES during pregnancy. Further studies confirmed the high occurrence of this clear-cell adenocarcinoma of the vagina and cervix in these women. Subsequent analysis has shown that the occurrence of this tumor varies between one in 1,000 to one in 10,000 of the daughters exposed to DES. Since the development of these tumors typically begins shortly after puberty, some hormonal stimulus, possibly a surge of the daughters own estrogens at the time puberty may trigger the development of this tumor. Unfortunately, this rare cancer is not the only side effect in DES-exposed daughters; other maladies include a variety of tissue changes and glandular enlargement in the cervix or vagina.

The data is conflicting as whether the mothers themselves have had a higher incidence of cancer. On the average, these women received between 10-12 grams of DES during pregnancy, which is a high dosage. There have been reports that these women have higher incidences of cancers of the breast, cervix, endometrium (lining of the uterus) and ovary than in a controlled population. However, the differences in occurrence are not considered statistically meaningful.

Determine if you were exposed to DES, either when pregnant or in utero, by checking with your doctor or mother. For example, a DES mother should try to verify from medical records the type of DES preparation she had taken, the dosage, when in pregnancy it was first administered, and the length of treatment. Women who had been exposed to DES should have this noted in their medical records, and should also have on-going evaluations to be sure no tumors are developing. The organs presumed to be at highest risk—and which should be checked most thoroughly—are the breasts and the reproductive tract. (For a complete explanation of self-examination, see Chapter 17).

Daughters of DES-exposed women should have a pelvic examination yearly, beginning at age 14. Pap smears and other evaluations are also recommended.

The long-term impact on sons of DES mothers is far less conclusive. There have been reports of increased occurrences of abnormalities of the reproductive organs and of testicular cancer, but the data is too fragmentary to be conclusive.

Since the daughters of DES mothers are just now beginning to enter the age zones—about 40-years-old—where the development of other tumors such as breast cancer usually occurs, these women should be particularly aware of changes in their breasts, even though no conclusive evidence yet exists that DES increases risk of such cancer in daughters.

Should DES daughters use oral contraceptives that contain estrogen and progesterone? For a variety of reasons the answer to this question is not yet known, but caution would favor the use of other birth control methods.

Estrogens have also been utilized to treat women with menopausal symptoms. Follow-up studies of these women have shown a four- to eight-fold increased risk of endometrial cancer. Furthermore, the higher the dosage of estrogen and the longer it was used, the higher the occurrence rate of endometrial cancer. Virtually all studies on this topic have suggested a cause and effect relationship between the use of estrogen at menopause and subsequent endometrial cancer. And, there has been a rising incidence of endometrial cancer in the United States. Fortunately, this excess risk of endometrial cancer diminishes after women stop using these hormones. Nevertheless, if you have been treated with estrogens for the relief of menopausal symptoms or for the prevention of osteoporosis, careful follow-up by a physician is mandatory.

Also, there is a possible relationship between menopausal estrogen use and the increased risk of breast cancer. Estrogen in the laboratory animal markedly increases the occurrence of breast cancer in susceptible strains of mice. However, the data in the human is far less clear. Some studies have shown an increase in breast cancer among women who have used estrogen at the menopause; others do not.

Oral Contraceptives

A number of years ago, the use of one type of sequential oral contraceptive (o.c.) was associated with an increased risk of cancer of the endometrium. Sequential oral contraceptives are those drugs which use estrogen alone during the first half of the monthly menstrual cycle, followed by a progesterone hormone in the second half. When sequential contraceptives are utilized, women are exposed to an unopposed estrogen action in the first half of the cycle. One sequential preparation which utilized unopposed estrogen for two days longer than other sequentials, and which also had the highest estrogen and lowest progesterone levels of any of these drugs, was eventually associated with an increase occurrence rate of endometrial cancer. Sequential o.c.'s are no longer prescribed or marketed.

There is evidence from a controlled study that the "combination" oral contraceptives, in which estrogens and progestins are given together, decreased by 50 percent the occurrence of cancer of the endometrium in comparison with women who have not used combination o.c.'s. This protective effect occurred in women who had used combination o.c.'s for at least 12 months, and persisted for at least 10 years after the women stopped taking the o.c.'s.

The Center for Disease Control estimates that the use of combination o.c.'s reduces the risk of developing cancer of the ovary. The risk decreased with increasing duration of use and remained low long after cessation of use.

However, the relation of oral contraceptives to the development of cancer of the cervix remains unsettled. Too many variables have been associated with studies of this type to have reached scientifically valid conclusions.

Also, an increased incidence of liver tumors among young women using oral contraceptives has been noted. The risk for users of the pill for 3-5 years was about 100 times greater than that of non-users. The risk appeared to be higher for users over the age of 30 and for users of pills containing higher dosages of estrogen and progestin. However, the absolute occurrence rate of these tumors is quite rare and the development of hepatomas— liver tumors—in women under age 30 is no more than three per 100,000 contraceptive users per year.

There have been a number of studies attempting to deter- mine the risk between o.c. use and breast cancer. The results are somewhat conflicting, but the consensus appears to be that there is no increase in breast cancer in women who have used the pill.

Androgens

Androgens are male sex hormones which, in addition to their masculinizing effect, also have an anabolic or tissue-building ac- tion and they are used to treat a variety of conditions. There have been reports that androgens, when used for the treatment of an unusual anemia called Fanconi anemia in young children, were associated with the development of cancer of the liver. Though it is difficult to scientifically link these hormones with liver tumors, the use of androgens or non-androgenic steroids by athletes at- tempting to improve muscular development and performance is ill-advised.

Alkylating Agents

Alkylating agents are a class of chemotherapeutic drugs in- cluding melphalan, cyclophosphamide and chlorambucil, used primarily in the treatment of malignant tumors. These drugs have been linked to an increased risk of developing a second cancer. For example, leukemia has developed in patients treated with melphalan or cyclophosphamide for multiple myeloma, a tumor arising in bone marrow. Patients treated for ovarian cancer with alkylating agents also show an increased risk in the development of leukemia. In the ovarian cancer and myeloma studies, it has been estimated that leukemia develops in 12-20 percent of patients who have been treated with alkalating agents and who survive 10 years. This represents a high incidence rate of leukemia.

Cyclophosphamide has also been related to an increased frequency of subsequent bladder cancer.

Immunosuppressive Agents

Immunosuppressive agents are drugs which are used to block or minimize the body's immunological responses to a foreign substance. They have been successful in prolonging the survival of transplanted organs such as the kidney. Follow-up studies have been performed on renal transplant patients who have received azathioprine and corticosteroids, both of which are immunosuppresive. In these patients, the risk of non-Hodgkin's lymphoma, a tumor of the lymph nodes, is increased 32-fold. This excess risk of lymphoma appeared within a short time after transplantation. Almost one-half of the lymphomas arose in the brain, which is a very unusual site for this type of tumor. Other types of cancer also developed in these immunosuppressed transplant patients.

Other Drugs

A number of other agents have been incriminated in the development of cancer in humans. Radioisotopes have been indicted in tumor induction in some patients. Radioactive phosphorous used in the treatment of polycythemia vera, a condition associated with increased red blood cells, prompts an increased risk of leukemia. Radium and mesothorium, which were previously utilized for the treatment of bone tuberculosis and other illnesses, produce a high rate of osteogenic sarcoma, a cancer of the bone.

Arsenicals have been shown to be associated with the increased occurrence of skin cancer. Arsenic was previously utilized in Fowlers solution, which was used for medicinal purposes. Analgesic mixtures containing phenacetin have been linked with a possible increase of the occurrence of cancer of the kidney.

Practical Implications

Certainly, when confronted with data of this type, the immediate reaction is to panic and to become frightened about *all* drug use. But remember, cancer is rarely caused by drugs. The overwhelming majority of drugs are correctly prescribed and are taken with great benefit by the patient. Only a miniscule percentage are associated with the possibility of tumor induction. This would occur when a potent drug with carcinogenic capacities is used at moderate dosage for a prolonged period of time. If in doubt, question your physician about possible adverse reactions of drug therapy, and remember, a drug should be used only when necessary and then at the minimal dosage and for the shortest period of time to achieve the desired results.

~ Thirteen ~

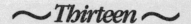

The Psychology of Cancer Prevention

Can emotional stress cause the development of cancer? Psychologists often cite a number of examples where cancer became apparent after an emotionally traumatic experience, such as the death of a loved one or the loss of a job. Actually, however, there is no proven cause-effect relationship between psychological stress and tumor induction; emotional reactions play no role in initiating the cellular changes which eventuate in cancer.

But, a person's state of mind can cause cancer. How can this apparent contradiction be true?

Cancer is sometimes precipitated by environmental factors resulting from habits which are established on a psychological basis. The classical example of behavioral influence on cancer induction is seen in smoking, which is associated with 25 percent of all cancers diagnosed in this country. Since 971,000 cancers developed this year in the United States, some 242,000 cancers are linked with people's "state of mind" toward tobacco. Sadly, the great majority of these cancers would be prevented if Americans could motivate themselves to stop smoking. .

Similarly, alcohol has been established as a culprit in most cancers of the intraoral tissues. Like smoking, excessive alcohol consumption has a psychological or behavioral basis. Drinking and smoking—often done concurrently—act synergistically to produce these cancers. Simple changes in a person's living patterns would eliminate or substantially reduce these neoplasms. Todd's history shows all too graphically the grim results which may await those who drink to excess and who smoke.

Why do people insist, in the face of all known medical evidence, on destroying their health by such habits? The specific answers to this question are, of course, unknown and presumably would vary with each individual.

However, some general observations can be made. A large part of the drinking and/or smoking problem seems to be habit formation. An individual may associate with people who smoke and drink and soon drifts into these habits himself. This peer-prompting is especially powerful with teenagers, many of whom fall into lifelong—and life-shortening—habits as youngsters. Though genetic or biochemical factors may be present in those who smoke or imbibe, such factors can certainly be overridden or controlled by a conscious decision by the individual to eliminate the habit. It is remarkable—and, in a way, disconcerting—to see the promptness, completeness and ease with which some patients discontinue smoking after being informed that they have developed a cancer. Typically, these are the selfsame individuals who had often protested that their "physical addiction" prevented them from ever stopping smoking. Unfortunately, for some persons, quitting comes a little too late.

Similarly, the liberalized social mores in this country have generated increased sexual permissiveness. As women begin intercourse at an earlier age, an almost certain result has been a striking increase in the numbers of young females with neoplastic changes in the cervix of the uterus. In later years, some of these women will develop cervical cancer.

Habits of a more innocent nature can also be associated with an increasing risk of cancer. The nation's commitment to sun-bathing, for example, will surely be producing more skin cancers in the future.

The essential thought behind these comments is that it is important to eliminate unhealthy patterns of living. Why self-destruct? Instead, eliminate unhealthy habits. I am not calling on you to attain monastic levels of discipline, but a modicum of self-restraint and a measure of common sense will promote a healthy life for you. Such moderation does not impair the joy in living; on the contrary, it heightens one's enjoyment by enhancing the body's physical condition. Eating a nutritious diet and avoiding an exces-sive caloric or animal fat intake is important. Appropriate exercise is beneficial for physical and emotional well-being.

Simply put, eliminating negative habits and maintaining pos-itive ones will improve your health and vitality and decrease your chances of developing cancer and other disease processes.

So, to a certain extent, the psychologists are right about the relationship between mind and cancer, but it is not the relation-ship they suggest. In many instances cancer does come from a state of the mind, and can often be prevented by the psychological commitment to healthy patterns of living.

You know what poor health practices are, as do practically all Americans. We are innundated with good advice about staying healthy, but too many times we don't act on it. What is needed is the courage to initiate a healthful pattern of living and to resist destructive peer pressure, whether it be to smoke in the high school locker room or to have the traditional martini at the busi-nessman's lunch. Common sense and self-discipline are indispen-sable for your health. You can improve your odds against cancer . . . if you want to.

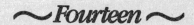

~ Fourteen ~

How to Detect Cancer Early

Certainly, our ideal goal is the prevention of cancer. Since many cancers are at least partially environmental in origin, prevention is possible in many cases. In fact, we can eliminate tens of thousands of cases of cancer in this country by simply adopting and maintaining healthful patterns of living.

Despite our best efforts, however, cancers will continue to develop for a number of reasons, some preventable and others totally unpreventable. Since all cancer cannot be prevented, then it is of critical importance to detect its presence at the earliest possible moment. In a number of organs, early detection is possible. It is difficult to define precisely what early detection is, since this varies widely depending upon the organ, the tumor's size, and whether or not it has spread.

Nevertheless, the concept of early detection is of utmost importance because it focuses your attention on a most important responsibility—that of discovering the tumor at the earliest possible moment. All of us—but particularly those in high-risk groups—should be sufficiently concerned with this objective to learn the simple steps to detect tumors early. This is particularly important for persons who are in high-risk groups. The high-risk individual is one who, for a number of reasons—either genetic or environmental—has an increased risk of developing cancer. Fortunately, this high-risk designation usually refers only to a specific organ and does not refer to an across-the-board increased risk in all organs. For example, the person at increased risk of developing cancer of the breast does not necessarily have an increased risk for melanoma.

Early detection improves your odds for beating the cancer. There is no doubt that cancer detected in its early stages has a significantly better prognosis than does cancer detected late in the course of its development. For example, cancer of the breast which is localized has a better-than-80 percent five-year cure rate, so the odds for Susan Webster are very good indeed. If the cancer, however, had spread to a distant organ, her five-year chance of survival would drop to only one chance in five and the cancer would probably cause her death during that period.

The prognosis for Todd McCormick is clearly poor. Though early cancer of the tongue can be cured by appropriate treatment in 80 percent of all cases, when the tumor spreads to the extent which Todd's has, the odds of survival drop dramatically.

Of lesser importance than the survival rate, but still important physically, emotionally and financially, is the fact that if cancer is detected early, treatment may be less aggressive or radical than is necessary for a more advanced tumor. An early cancer of the vocal cord, for example, is treatable by either irradiation therapy or by a modest surgical excision; both offer excellent cure rates with minimal disability. If, however, this same cancer involved wider areas of the larynx and the adjacent neck, a much more formidable treatment approach must be undertaken, possibly involving rather massive surgery of the neck area coupled with irradiation therapy. Under these circumstances, the larynx would be removed and normal speech would be lost. Talking would be accomplished by esophogeal speech or by the creation of an artificial opening between the windpipe and the pharynx.

The adverse effects of late cancer detection are many, including diminished survival rates and steep costs in pain, emotional suffering, loss of body parts and negative self-image. Of lesser concern, but important nonetheless, is the economic havoc late cancer detection can wreak on patient and family.

Pre-Symptomatic Detection of Cancer

Most cancers begin in one area of the body and remain there for varying but significant periods of time before metastasizing. Contrary to popular belief not all cancer cells divide with great rapidity. But, once cancer cells begin to divide, their growth is inexorable. This means that for varying and unknown intervals of time, the cancer remains localized. For example, a cancer of the breast may require several years to grow from one cell to one centimeter—half an inch in size. At this phase of its growth, the cancer would be highly curable.

Our objective, therefore, is to detect cancers before they grow to the point where they produce symptoms; this is known as pre-symptomatic detection.

An important objective of this book is to offer to you practical, reasonable and relatively inexpensive ways to detect cancer in an early phase. Such detection can be achieved by periodic self-examinations and by evaluations by a health professional. Examination of healthy individuals has been endorsed as an excellent health strategy by organizations with impeccable scientific credentials. For example, the importance of such "well person" exams has been cited and endorsed by the Council on Scientific Affairs of the American Medical Association, the American Cancer Society, the Canadian Task Force on Periodic Health Examination, the Institute of Medicine and the American College of Physicians. The concensus is clear—periodic examination of healthy persons is beneficial.

As might be expected, there are differences of opinion regarding the specifics of such health check-ups and the intervals at

73

which they should be performed. For example, the American Cancer Society recommends a Pap test on a three-year basis after two consecutive negative annual exams. Once the "prevalent" cancer population—those who have cervical cancer—has been screened out by two negative annual examinations, the occurrence rate of invasive cancer of the cervix is extremely low. In fact, thousands of women must be screened to find a single invasive cancer. Clearly, the cost efficiency of annual or bi-annual exams is not good. Not all medical opinon is unanimous on this point, however; most gynecologists recommend an annual Pap test.

~ Fifteen ~

Guidelines for Cancer Detection in Asymptomatic Persons

The single most effective way to detect an early cancer is to have periodical check-ups with a physican or a health professional. Since these are examinations of asymptomatic persons, they should occur on a scheduled basis even though no symptoms are present. The best chance to beat cancer is when the tumor hasn't grown enough to produce any symptoms. Your evaluation should consist of a medical history and a physical examination oriented toward tumor detection. Simple tests may be performed. Counselling in good health habits should be offered.

Guidelines for these examinations are presented in the accompanying table. Remember, these are guidelines only and can and should be modified by individual circumstances, including your age, risk factors and emotional makeup. They are reasonable steps for a prudent person to pursue but there must be flexibility

75

in their utilization. Such risk factors as a family history of cancer, excessive drinking, smoking, DES exposure in-utero, blue-eyed, fair-skinned complexion, etc. are all characteristics which increase your likelihood of developing specific cancers. All of these factors must be considered in making the decision about frequency of examination.

The cancer history, taken by a health professional, should elicit information on the risk factors for cancer, many of which have been outlined. Additionally, inquiries should be made about symptoms which might suggest the presence of an early cancer.

A physical examination for tumor detection would include careful evaluation of the skin, the head and neck, lymph nodes, abdominal palpation, and digital exam of the rectum. In men, examination of the testes and prostate should be done; women should have breast and pelvic examinations with Pap smear. Other simple tests such as blood pressure could be done quite easily. While this has no immediate bearing on cancer detection, it does uncover asymptomatic hypertension.

A slide for occult blood in the stool may detect a pre-symptomatic cancer of the gastrointestinal tract. Sigmoidoscopy or inspection of the lower colon can also pick up small tumors of this area. Mammography detects cancer of the breast earlier and with greater efficiency than physical examination and decreases the mortality rates of breast cancer.

Counselling is a vital component of this cancer detection process. The health professional should make recommendations for improving the person's pattern of living and give instruction and encouragement in the performance of self-examination. Such counselling unquestionably enhances the patient's awareness of good health practices.

Most of these procedures and studies can be done by properly trained nurses and paramedical personnel. This would increase the efficiency and cost-effectiveness of these procedures. Such periodic evaluations could be made a part of the fringe benefit programs of major offices, factories, unions, etc. Even if your insurance or office or union doesn't cover preventive exams, and you have to pay out-of-pocket, these tests promote your health and peace of mind and they are worth it.

76

Special Techniques for Early Diagnosis

Techniques which permit early tumor detection and diagnosis for cancers of the colon and uterus are so effective that they warrant detailed descriptions. You should know something about them because they play important roles in safeguarding your health.

Colon and Rectum

One hundred and forty-five thousand new cases of cancer of the colon and the rectum developed in the United States this year. These diseases, which may be considered as one, are so common that their combined incidence ranked second only to that of lung cancer. Colo-rectal cancer causes 60,000 deaths annually. However, screening and other diagnostic techniques can improve mortality figures.

Certain risk factors are associated with the development of this cancer. Familial polyposis of the colon is a hereditary disorder which occurs in both sexes and is characterized by the presence of innumerable polyps in the colon and rectum. Initially, these polyps are benign but have a tendency to become malignant. These cancers occur at an age which is younger than the usual colon cancer. Colon cancers develop about 15 years after the onset of the symptoms of polyposis.

Unfortunately, the most impressive feature of this disease is that 100 percent of patients with familial polyposis will develop cancer. They develop this early in life. The average age of death from cancer in multiple polyposis patients is 42 years. Comparatively, the average age of death for patients with colon of the cancer in the general population is 67.

Chronic ulcerative colitis is another risk factor. This disease of unknown causation affects the colon and the rectum primarily of younger people and produces an inflammation of the mucosa or surface lining of the large bowel. Symptoms of this condition include diarrhea, bleeding and pain; a high percentage of patients with chronic ulcerative colitis will develop cancer of the colon.

Since colo-rectal cancer is primarily found in Western society, it may be related to environmental factors, such as dietary habits. Some investigators believe that high fat and low fiber diets may be a causative factor.

Early diagnosis is seldom made if reliance is placed on waiting for the appearance of symptoms because the colon and rectum are quite capacious organs which, unfortunately, can adjust well to the presence of even large tumor masses. Symptoms are produced only when the tumor obstructs the colon, or when a sufficient amount of bleeding occurs to attract the attention of the patient. Usually, these symptoms connote moderately far-advanced disease. It is, however, possible to detect these cancers much earlier in their genesis by testing the stool for occult, or hidden, blood. Benign and malignant tumors and other conditions frequently cause varying degrees of bleeding into the stool. This amount of blood is so small it may escape detection by the eye, but its presence is uncovered by a simple chemical test.

Commercially available guaiac slides are utilized to check the stool for the presence of occult blood. This test is done at home by smearing minute amounts of stool with a wooden spatula on the slides on three consecutive days. The slides are then forwarded to a physician or laboratory for testing. To increase the accuracy of this test, avoid taking aspirin for a week or so prior to obtaining these stool specimens since aspirin can irritate the gastro-intestinal tract and cause minor degrees of bleeding which cause a false positive reading. Similarly, a red-meat free diet and the avoidance of Vitamin C also increase the tests validity. These latter steps of avoiding aspirin, Vitamin C and red meat are required if a previous test has been read as positive. Please remember that positive results on this test are usually not due to cancer but from some other cause such as hemorrhoids. Nevertheless, a positive result for occult blood demands a further evaluation to determine the precise cause of bleeding.

The next aid to the pre-symptomatic detection of colo-rectal cancer is a rectal examination by a physician. This examination reveals whether or not a tumor mass is present in the rectum. In men, the prostate gland can also be examined by this maneuver.

If blood has been found in the stool, a sigmoidoscopy should be performed. This examination should be done over age 40 even if blood is not present. In this exam, the physician inserts a lighted metal tube to inspect the lower 25 centimeters of the rectum and the colon. Even small cancers are readily apparent with this magnified viewing system. More recently, a flexible sigmoidoscope has been devised which allows the examination of the colon to higher levels.

If blood is present in the stool and rectal exam and sigmoidoscopy do not reveal its source, further evaluation by X-ray studies and endoscopy are performed. In colonoscopy a flexible instrument is inserted into the rectum which can traverse and inspect the entire length of the large bowel around to the cecum in the right side. Removal of polyps and biopsies of tumors can be performed with this instrument. The barium enema can be utilized to study the full length of the colon. In skillful hands, this can reveal quite small tumors. If no tumors of the colon and rectum are discovered, the upper gastro-intestinal tract, including the esophagus, should be evaluated.

Though colo-rectal cancer does not produce early symptoms, it can be diagnosed in an early stage by checking the stool for occult blood, by digital rectal examination and by sigmoidoscopy. The encouraging feature about this diagnostic attack is that the cancers detected earlier in the course of their development have an appreciable better prognosis than tumors which grow large enough to produce symptoms. Furthermore, in addition to detecting cancers these tests will detect benign polyps of the lower colon and rectum. These polyps may or may not turn into cancer; all authorities agree that these polyps can and should be removed.

Early cancer of the colon and rectum can be detected by these techniques. If you have this cancer and it is detected before it produces symptoms, your prognosis will be greatly improved.

Cancers of the Uterus

Cancer develops in both the body, or upper part, of the uterus and in the cervix or lower portion. Although located in the same organ, these cancers differ so appreciably in causation and in clinical behavior that they must be considered separately.

Cancer of the cervix developed in 13,000 American women this year and killed 6,800 women. Clearly, this graphically illustrates that though there has been a 70 percent drop in deaths from this cancer during the last 40 years, it is still a major health problem in our country. The cervix is one of only two potential cancer sites which have shown marked improvement in mortality rates. Stomach cancer is the other tumor which has diminished because the occurrence of this tumor has been falling steadily for unknown reasons.

However, the cause of the decline in the death rate for cervical cancer is clear and unequivocal; it is the result of the Papanicolau test, more commonly known as the Pap smear, which detects the earliest manifestations of this disease. The Pap smear is unique because it alone allows detection of a cancer in the very earliest stage of its development, before it has begun to invade. When detected in this phase, the disease is easily treated by simple means, often in the physician's office, and it is almost completely curable. If similar early-warning techniques were available for other organs in the body, cancer would no longer be the scourge it is today.

To understand the report on a Pap test, you must know something about the cells of the cervix. Normally, this structure is lined by cells, called squamous cells, which look flattened when viewed under the microscope. Layers of these cells are piled atop each other like flattened stones in a wall to produce a tissue called the epithelium, the surface membrane of the cervix.

Under the influence of a number of factors, the squamous cells of the lower one-third of the epithelium undergo a transition into abnormal cells, assuming the appearance of tumor or neoplastic cells. During this process, known as dysplasia, these abnormal cells are termed dysplastic cells.

If such cells occupy only the lower one-third of the epithelium, the condition is referred to as mild dysplasia, also designated by the more formidable term of cervical intra-epithelial neoplasia, Grade 1 (CIN Grade 1). If the dysplastic cells continue their upward migration from the base of the epithelium and occupy two-thirds of the thickness of this structure, this more serious condition is termed as moderate dysplasia or CIN Grade 2. Severe dysplasia, or CIN Grade 3, occurs when the cells reach almost to the surface of the cervix. When the entire epithelium, which measures about two-tenths of a millimeter—or about the thickness of this page—is occupied by these abnormal cells, the lesion is diagnosed as a carcinoma in-situ, which is also designated as CIN Grade 3.

These changes are precursors of invasive cancer of the cervix. This belief is supported by the simultaneous presence of carcinoma in-situ and invasive cancer, and by the fact that invasive cancer frequently occurs in patients who are not treated for cervical intra-epithelial neoplasia.

The next stage in the development of cancer of the cervix occurs when these neoplastic cells begin to invade the stroma, which is the tissue underlying the epithelium. When this infiltration occurs to such a minor degree that it can be detected only under the microscope, it is called microinvasive carcinoma. This represents the transition period between carcinoma in-situ, which presents no threat of metastases, and an invasive cancer that may spread from the stroma to distant locations and can ultimately result in the death of the patient.

The final phase of the development of cervical cancer is designated as invasive carcinoma. At this stage, cancer can be seen to be invading into and destroying the cervix.

The development of cancer of the cervix stretches across a continuum of changes, beginning with some mildly abnormal cells in the depths of the epithelium and eventuating with invasive cancer.

This is not, however, an inexorable process. Dysplasia, which is a benign condition, takes one of three courses; these are regression, persistance, or progression to invasive cancer. Though it is uncertain what percentage of these lesions will follow each respective course, if they are detected early in their development, these benign conditions can be eradicated and their possible progression to a cancer of the cervix will halted.

The epochal importance of the Pap smear is that it can detect these abnormal cellular changes in the cervix in the very earliest stages of their development. This test, named after its discoverer, Dr. George Papanicolou, consists of a microscopic inspection of cervical cells. These cells are collected by a number of techniques, including wiping the surface of the cervix with a wooden spatula, or by aspiration. After the cells are smeared upon a glass slide and stained, they are examined by a cytologist to detect the changes characteristic of dysplasia or cancer. The Pap smear has a very impressive 95 percent accuracy rate in detecting cervical cancer.

Dysplasia of the cervix is a potential pre-cursor of cancer and may have few or no overt symptoms. Detection depends upon screening asymptomatic women by the Pap test. Abnormal smears require further diagnostic procedures.

Though the mortality rate of cervical cancer has dropped dramatically, the increasing use of cytologic screening has uncovered dysplasias and microinvasive cancer in ever-younger groups of patients. Previously, the median age at diagnosis of carcinoma in-situ was about 40 years; in some studies this has now fallen to 28, and it is not unusual to see teenagers with significant CIN lesions. So, while mortality rates for cancer of the cervix have been declining because of the detection capabilities of the Pap smear, there has been a concurrent increase in the numbers of young women developing neoplastic changes of the cervix.

This unfortunate phenomenon is attributable to changing, liberalized, sexual mores. Using simple extrapolation, it is apparent that we will see a large increase in the numbers of women suffering from neoplastic cervical disease. Therefore, vigorous surveillance of this population is essential to prevent the tragic consequences of invasive cancer. The deadly course of this disease is readily evident in such impoverished regions as Latin America, where cancer of the cervix is the most common form of malignancy in women and has achieved endemic proportions.

Other diagnostic tools have been developed to aid the physician in treating this tumor. When abnormal Pap smears indicate changes in the cervix, a colposcopy, the inspection of the cervix through an instrument which gives a magnified steroscopic view of the surface epithelium, is required. This examination allows detection of otherwise invisible sites from which the abnormal cells are being shed and permits accurate biopsy of the cervix to establish the nature and extent of the abnormality.

If a grossly evident tumor or ulceration of the cervix is present, biopsy can be performed without colposcopy.

Because of its preventive—and potentially life-saving—role, cytologic screening is a mandatory part of any effective cancer prevention program. Women should be screened regularly once they begin sexual activity, no matter what their age. This preventive step allows detection of early intra-epithelial lesions which can lead to cancer of the cervix; these precancerous lesions are easier to eradicate and treat than invasive carcinoma.

These diagnostic procedures can be performed on an outpatient basis. However, further diagnostic tests which are performed in the hospital may sometimes be necessary. There, tissue can be removed from the inner aspect of the cervical canal by a technique known as conization, or cone biopsy.

Endometrial Cancer

More common than cervical cancer is endometrial cancer, which arises in the inner lining of the body of the uterus. It is more common than cancer of the cervix and affected 35,000 women in our country this year while claiming 2,900 lives. Primarily a disease of post-menopausal women, its most common symptom is post-menopausal bleeding.

A number of factors are associated with an increased risk of developing cancer of the endometrium, including obesity, hypertension or high blood pressure, diabetes and infertility. Other conditions which may be associated include irregular menses, failure to ovulate, a pre-cancerous change in the endometrium termed adenomatous hyperplasia, and prolonged use of estrogen. In contradistinction to cervical cancer, which is manifested mostly in women of lower socio-economic classes, endometrial carcinoma appears most frequently in women of higher socio-economic status.

The incidence of endometrial cancer is increasing in this country, though the cause of this rise is uncertain. It may be related to an aging population, obesity, or the increased administration of estrogens for menopausal symptoms, which increases the risk of developing endometrial cancer four-fold. This causal relationship to estrogen imbalance has been further suggested by the fact that endometrial cancer frequently accompanies ovarian tumors, which secrete estrogen. Conversely, endometrial cancer is quite infrequent in patients who have had a previous ovariectomy.

Unfortunately, the Pap smear, which is highly accurate in the detection of cervical cancer, is only about 65 percent efficient in detecting cancers of endometrium. A possible warning sign of development of this cancer is the presence of adenomatous hyperplasia, a proliferation of the cells of the endometrium which, although benign, may be a pre-cancerous process. Adenomatous hyperplasia is most commonly seen in menopausal women, particularly those with abnormal bleeding. Adenomatous hyperplasia may be treated with the administration of progestins, a hormonal substance. This is frequently done in younger women who wish to avoid hysterectomy and have children.

Improvements in the cure rates for endometrial cancer can be achieved by identifying high-risk patients and following them carefully, especially at the menopause. Peri-menopausal or post-menopausal women who develop abnormal bleeding should have tissue evaluation to rule out the presence of a tumor.

The physician has a number of techniques for detecting early endometrial cancer, including Pap smears and the use, upon appropriate indication, of biopsies of the endometrial cavity for histologic study. This procedure can be performed on an outpatient basis. If further evaluation is necessary, the patient may be admitted to the the hospital briefly for a D&C—dialation and curettage—a scraping of the lining of the uterus to obtain tissue for analyses.

The key to improving the odds against developing any uterine cancer lies with the woman herself. Visit your physician for appropriate care particularly if you are at high risk for developing these cancers and, more importantly, be alert to any abnormal bleeding, which is cause for an immediate visit to your physician.

Guidelines for Cancer Detection in Asymptomatic Persons

Procedure or Test	Age	Frequency
Cancer History and Physical		
Skin	20	annually
Intra-oral	40	annually
Neck	20	annually
Breast	20	annually
Nodes	20	annually
Abdomen	40	annually
Genitalia	20	annually
Prostate	40	annually
Rectal	40	annually
Pelvic	20	annually
Pap smear	20*	annually
Sigmoidoscopy	40	every 2 years
Stool occult blood	40	annually
Mammogram	40**	see footnote
Urinalysis	40	annually
Chest X-ray	40***	see footnote

*or younger, if sexually active

**age 40 base line, then every 2 years; over 50 every 1-2 years or as determined by risk factors

***as determined by risk factors; annually for heavy smoker

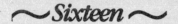

~ Sixteen ~

Examine Yourself for Cancer

An annual check-up with your physician is an effective way to improve your chances of detecting early cancer. But if a tumor begins to manifest itself shortly after your annual visit, the time lag before your next appointment may be too long. Since it is impractical to go to the doctor every few months for evaluations, you must examine yourself for cancer.

Self-detection of tumors is not only possible, but relatively simple. It requires that you know the clincal appearances of cancer and that you commit yourself to performing monthly examinations. Selecting and sticking with a particular day—such as your birthdate—for these examinations makes them easier to do faithfully. Cancer of the skin, intraoral tissue, thyroid gland, salivary glands, lymph nodes, breast and testis are often detected through self-examination. If you do your self-examination monthly, you will become familiar with the appearance and feel of your own tissues while they are healthy; consequently, if a tumor does develop, you should be able to detect it at the earliest possible moment.

A word of advice: Most persons are able to examine themselves without undue emotional stress or anxiety. Most, in fact, find a normal examination to be a reassuring exercise. However, some people cannot perform self-detection procedures with equanimity. If you are one of those individual who is made unduly nervous by this practice, you are better off not doing it.

Don't become alarmed by your initial self-examination. You may discover lumps that are normal body structures, and erroneously conclude that you have cancer. If you are worried you have detected cancer in your initial self-examination, go to your doctor for a professional evaluation. In the great majority of cases, he will allay your fears.

After your initial few self-examinations, you will be able to recognize what is normal and detect a pathologic condition.

Self-examination is no guarantee that you will detect an early tumor. Despite your best efforts, it may not be detectable, or you may miss it on your examination. Even experienced physicians can miss tumors. Nevertheless, self-examination is an important aide to early cancer detection. Make it work for you.

Cancer of the Skin

There are three types of cancer of the skin: basal cell carcinoma, squamous cell carcinoma and melanoma. Basal cell carcinoma is not an aggressive tumor and, if detected and treated, is curable in almost 100 percent of cases. Only neglected basal cell cancer can produce death, and this does occasionally occur. Squamous cell cancer is slightly more aggressive but, again, with early detection, the great majority of these tumors are cured. Malignant melanoma, more commonly referred to as melanoma, is a significantly more aggressive cancer which is associated with substantial mortality rates. Basal cell and squamous cell cancers, because they are so similar, will be discussed together; melanoma will be presented separately.

Basal and squamous cell carcinomas, also referred to as non-melanoma skin cancers, are the most common cancers in the human body. Each year, an estimated 500,000 cases of this disease develop in the United States. Fortunately, only about 2,000 patients per year die of these types of cancer. Unfortunately, no one should die of these tumors. These skin cancers, because they occur on an external organ, are easily inspected and palpated. They should be detected early and cured in all cases. Additionally, early detection mandates less drastic treatment and cosmetic results are enhanced. How pervasive is non-melanoma skin cancer? About half of all people who reach 65 years of age will have had at least one such cancer.

Basal cell cancer is the most common form of skin cancer and occurs primarily in individuals exposed to prolonged or intense sunlight, especially in those with light eyes, light hair and a fair complexion. It typically manifests itself on sun-exposed surfaces. Metastases (spread to other organs) of these tumors are extremely uncommon.

Here is how you can inspect your skin for these cancers. First, you must be familiar with their appearance and characteristic patterns. One of these, known as nodulo-ulcerative basal cell cancer, is characterized by the elevation of a tumor nodule with central ulceration of the skin, surrounded by a raised waxy or "pearly" border. Another type of basal cell is called the superficial basal cell cancer and is characterized by a slightly elevated placque formation. It will often have a crust or scab on its surface.

The squamous cell cancer has a variety of appearances, ranging from an elevated mass to a punched-out type of ulceration. These cancers can, if neglected, metastasize to regional lymph nodes and sometimes to distant organs through the blood stream.

The essential feature to watch for in detecting either of these lesions is the presence of destruction of the normal surface of the skin, resulting in ulceration which is characterized by weeping or even bleeding. If you should see this type of ulceration, seek medical aid. These cancers are primarily located on sun-exposed surfaces and are quite common about the head and neck area.

Examine your skin once a month. The skin of the front of your body is easily inspected. But remember the skin of the back is frequently the site of cancer. You can check your back by using hand-held and wall mirrors, or else have a family member or friend check the skin surfaces of your back which you cannot see.

Any tumor nodule or any lesion which fails to heal, scabs, crusts over and then falls off and begins to re-bleed warrants your attention. One problem with detecting these skin cancers is that they develop rather slowly and you can become accustomed to them without noticing their presence, particularly since they cause no pain. They are often neglected. Consequently, conscientious monthly examinations are recommended.

Although basal and squamous cell cancers have excellent cure rates, be aware of one exception to this rule. Occasionally, squamous cell cancer will develop in a pre-existing burn scar or in a scar resulting from chronic inflammation. When this happens the cancer can be much more aggressive and may be fatal. As a result, pay particular attention to skin changes around such burns, scars and old draining wounds.

Malignant melanoma is a tumor of distinctly different character. An estimated 26,000 people developed melanoma this year in this country and about 5,800 die from it. Disturbingly, the incidence of melanoma is climbing sharply at about the rate of 8 percent a year. Our cure rates for melanoma are far from ideal. However, the vast majority of these deaths are preventable because the cancer arises in an externally situated organ, the skin, and should be detected early.

Most melanomas arise in pre-existing, benign pigmented moles, also called nevi. Nevi are extremely common in the Caucasian population; each individual has about 15 nevi. Fortunately, only one nevus in many thousands develops into a melanoma. But because individuals become so accustomed to the presence of their nevi, they pay them little or no attention. Consequently, when these nevi turn into melanomas, even though they signal this transformation to cancer by an alteration in their appearance, the changes are often overlooked by the patient.

There are a number of warning signs signaling the malignant change. Normally, the nevus or mole is tan or brown and looks much like all other moles. The mole is round and there are clearly defined borders between it and the surrounding skin. It is flat or slightly elevated and usually relatively small in size, measuring less than five millimeters—about the diameter of a pencil eraser. Moles or nevi are usually located on sun-exposed surfaces above the waist—particularly on the face and arms. Conversely, the scalp, the breast and the buttocks are not commonly involved.

When a mole manifests a change in color—particularly when it becomes red, white, blue, black or mottled shades of brown and black—it may be undergoing a malignant change. If a mole undergoes an increase in surface diameter or or if it changes outline, especially with the development of irregular or notched borders, a cancer may be developing. Other characteristics in a nevus signaling malignant transformation include scaliness, erosion, seeping of blood, ulceration, or the development of a tumor nodule. Also, if the nevus becomes elevated from a previously flat condition or if there is an extension of pigment from the nevus out into the surrounding skin, melanoma may be developing.

Recently, a new type of nevus or mole has been recognized which has been termed a dysplastic nevus. These nevi have a slightly different appearance from the common mole. They may have additional coloration in the form of black or reddish pigment and their borders may be notched. They are usually bigger than the other types of moles and they frequently number more than 100 per patient. The significant fact about these nevi is that there is a greater chance of them developing into a melanoma than there is with a common garden variety mole.

In brief, any change in appearance—size, color, consistency ulceration or elevation—in a pre-existing mole or nevus should bring you promptly to your physician.

Inspect your skin surfaces now so that you know what your moles look like. Then, if any of them do develop into tumors, you will detect them on your monthly exam.

Remember that the overwhelming majority of pigmented skin lesions that you have will not be melanomas; most, in fact, will not even be moles. Admittedly, it is difficult, even for the physician, to distinguish between the benign nevus and melanoma. The key, once again, is change in appearance. If this develops, seek medical attention promptly.

Though it is difficult to give a scientifically-based estimate as to how much higher the cure rate would be with early detection of melanoma, it's reasonable to say it would improve by 25 percent.

Death by skin cancer is avoidable. All you have to do is inspect your skin and feel its surface, and seek medical opinion at the first sign of change.

Breast

Cancer of the breast is the most common cancer in women. In fact, its incidence in women is so frequent that it is the third most common cancer in men and women together, and is exceeded only by lung and colo-rectal cancer. This year, 130,000 new cases of breast cancer were diagnosed in the United States, meaning that one of every 10 women will develop cancer of the breast. Also, this year 41,000 women died of this disease, making it the second leading cause of death from cancer in women. Only lung cancer kills more women.

Incidence rates of breast cancer are increasing in the United States as well as in Europe. Diagnostic efforts are important, therefore to detect breast cancer earlier and improve prognosis.

Risk Factors

The most significant risk factor in the development of cancer of the breast is age. The incidence begins increasing around age 30 and progresses to very high rates by age 70.

Interestingly, the incidence of breast cancer varies throughout the world. The rates are high in Western and industrialized countries such as the United States, Canada, Europe and Australia; intermediate rates are noted in Eastern and Southern European countries; the rates are low in Asia, Latin America and Africa. Genetic factors play some role in this variation but environmental factors such as reproductive practices, socio-economic status and diet are of more significance, because women born in countries with a low incidence of breast cancer manifest an increase in rates after they migrate to the United States. While the rates in these immigrants are higher than those of women in the country of their birth, they are still below United States rates. Daughters of European immigrants reach American rates within one generation; Asian women appear to require more than one generation.

Undoubtedly, a family history of breast cancer predisposes a woman to the development of this condition. The risk of women whose mothers or sisters have had breast cancer is two- to fourfold higher than that of the at-large population. This risk is magnified if more than one close relative—mother or sisters—had breast cancer. Furthermore, if the disease developed in a relative who was pre-menopausal, the predisposition is even greater. And if the disease developed in both breasts of a close relative, then there is an even more severe degree of risk.

For many years, we have known that marital status affects the occurrence of breast cancer. As long ago as 1700, it was recorded that nuns had an excess risk of cancer of the breast; this was attributed to their celibacy. Now, it appears that the protective influence of marriage is due to the more common occurrence of pregnancy in married women than in their unmarried counterparts. This protective influence is primarily concentrated in a lower rate of cancer after the menopause; among women age 35-45 years, breast cancer rates do not differ significantly by marital status.

Numerous studies have demonstrated an inverse relationship between pregnancy and breast cancer; cancer of the breast is significantly less in women who have multiple pregnancies than in women who have never been pregnant. In fact, women with a full-term pregnancy before age 20 experience only one-third the risk of developing breast cancer than women whose first childbirth occurred after age 35. Other analyses show that births subsequent to the first have little or no additional protective impact. Therefore, the reduced risk previously attributed to women with multiple pregnancies is apparently due to their first pregnancy usually occurring early in life. Furthermore, this protective effect from early first pregnancy appears to be confined to full-term births. Pregnancies ending in abortion or miscarriage apparently do not reduce subsequent risk of breast cancer.

This data suggests that a breast cancer-inducing factor occurs with the onset of menses in the adolescent female. This factor is minimized or eliminated by the first full-term pregnancy. The duration of this cancer-causing factor is important in determining breast cancer risk and would explain the decreased occurrence of breast cancer in women who deliver full-term infants early in life.

Another fact related to the frequency of breast cancer is length of active reproductive life. The early onset of menses and late menopause have both been associated with increasing occurrence of breast cancer. Conversely, an artificial menopause by removal of the ovaries is associated with a substantial reduction in breast cancer risk when performed before age 40.

Lactation was thought to have a beneficial effect in preventing breast cancer; however, more recent studies suggest that this beneficial effect is due primarily to an early first pregnancy.

The existence of a previous cancer of the breast in the individual herself is another risk factor. If such a cancer has occurred, the patient is at a substantial increase in risk of developing a cancer in the opposite breast. Breast cancer is appreciably more common in women of upper socioeconomic groups, probably because early pregnancy is less common in this group of women. Eating habits—particularly a high caloric, high fat diet—may also play a role in this relationship.

Finally, certain types of fibrocystic disease of the breast increase breast cancer risk. This condition, which is characterized by nodular thickenings and cysts in the breast, increases the possibility of developing breast cancer by about three-fold.

Susan Webster obviously had been at an increased risk of developing cancer of the breast, a fact which she realized. She was of a higher socioeconomic group and enjoyed the dietary patterns which this status allows. She had never been pregnant. Further increasing her risks were the facts that her mother had had cancer of the breast and that she herself had fibrocystic disease. To her credit, Susan realized these increased risks and took special precautions. She had periodic examinations by a physician and, most importantly, had performed monthly breast self-examinations. This habit enabled her to detect her breast cancer at the earliest possible moment.

Please remember that all risk factors must be kept in proper perspective. For example, if the breast cancer occurrence rate in all women is about 10 percent, your chances, if you have an aggressive form of fibrocystic disease, are increased three-fold—to about 30 percent. This is a definite increase, but remember that about 70 percent of women with such fibrocystic disease will not develop breast cancer. Here, the odds are on your side.

Also, we are dealing here with statistics for large populations which say nothing about the outlook for you as an individual.

So, again, it is important for you to keep all of this in perspective. However, if you do have one or more risk factors, take prudent care of yourself by following these suggestions for self- and professional examinations. Don't panic about your prospects, because the odds are clearly in your favor.

Breast Self-Examination

Usually, breast cancers are first detected by the woman herself. However, in most instances, the detection occurred by chance and not as a part of a regular breast self-examination program. Consequently, most of the tumors detected by chance are larger than those detected in systematic regular examination programs and have a less optimistic prognosis. Unfortunately, most women do not examine their breasts routinely, and many women who say they do perform breast self-examination (BSE), do so improperly. Their self-examinations are infrequent, occurring at three or four month intervals. They are usually hurried, lasting only a number of seconds to a minute or so. Finally, the technique of the examination itself is poor.

To improve your odds against cancer it is mandatory that you perform a frequent, thorough, systematic and technically correct examination of your breasts.

BSE should be performed monthly. For a pre-menopausal woman, the best time is the second or third day after the onset of menses. At this time, the breasts will be less engorged and a tumor mass more easily palpable. Women who are post-menopausal should arbitrarily select one day in the month; their birthdate or some other date that is easily remembered.

Examination consists of three phases. In the first, the breasts are examined while bathing. Friction between fingers and breasts is decreased when the skin surface is wet and makes it easier to detect small breast tumors.

The second technique is to examine the breasts in a large mirror. Inspect the contour of the breasts to ascertain if they are basically symmetric in appearance. Breasts normally differ somewhat in size, but their overall appearance should be similar. Look closely for the presence of a visible mass or fullness, which could indicate an underlying tumor. Also, inspect the nipples for evidence of scaling and/or bleeding or discharge. Look to see if there is dimpling or retraction of the skin. This may indicate the presence of an underlying cancer which is pulling the skin in. Retraction or inversion of the nipple may also be a manifestation of cancer; some women, however, have always had inverted nipples on a congenital basis, and this is no cause for alarm. Next, raise your arms above your head and inspect the contour of the breasts to see if there is any change, such as the appearance of a mass, dimpling or a retraction.

The third phase of the examination is to lie on the bed and palpate the breasts with the pads at the ends of your four fingers (Fig. 1). Use the right hand for the left breast and vice versa. This examination should take place in a systematic fashion to assure that no area of the breast is missed.

Imagine the breast as a clock. Begin your examination at the top of the breast in the 12 o'clock position. With a firm but gentle motion, sweep the fingertips down along the 12 o'clock radius to the nipple. Repeat this several times. Then, along the same axis, gently pat the same area. Repeat two or three times. Then move to the 1 o'clock position and so forth, until you complete the entire breast examination in this same way. Remember also to examine the portion of the breast underneath the nipple and the areola and to check for the presence of any tumor masses in the armpit, or axilla.

Undoubtedly, breast self-examination can detect early breast cancers. However, there are difficulties with this examination which unfortunately are usually not mentioned in BSE promotional literature. For example, the breasts may be very large, making the examination difficult. Also, some women have, by

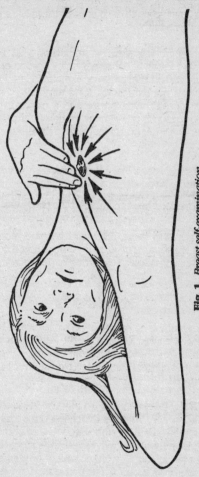

Fig. 1. Breast self-examination.

nature, a nodular pattern to the breast. This makes it difficult to detect small tumors. Nevertheless, most women will, with repeated examinations, become familiar with what their breasts feel like. Then, if a new growth does appear, they have a good chance of detecting it promptly.

Another confusing situation regarding BSE is that much breast tissue is located in the upper outer portion of each breast, extending up toward the axilla, or armpit. Occasionally, women will mistake this normal breast finding for a tumor. To distinguish between normal breast architecture and a tumor in this vicinity, check for the presence of a similar finding on the opposite side. If both upper outer quadrants feel essentially the same, it is likely not a tumor.

A breast cancer feels like a firm or hard lump with a difficult-to-define outline. If you detect a unique or dominant mass in the breast, report to your physician or clinic for further evaluation. Reassuringly, 80 percent—or more—of such masses are benign.

As you perform more BSE's and become more and more familiar with the texture of your breasts, you will consider your monthly self-examination a reassuring experience.

Mammography

Mammography is an examination of the breast by X-ray. Usually, two views are taken of each breast—a side, or mediolateral view, and an up-and-down, or cranio-caudad, view. With mammography, breast cancers can be detected at a very early stage in their development.

In the X-ray, breast cancer usually reveals itself as a tumor with irregular borders. Another indication is the existence of fine calcifications, which are tiny stones in one area of the breast. Not infrequently, mammograms will reveal the presence of a tumor which cannot be palpated by either patient or physician because of its small size or its location. For that reason, the mammogram is an important part of the detection process for asymptomatic women.

The American Cancer Society, in conjunction with the National Cancer Institute, has conducted an extensive five-year breast cancer demonstration project. In this study of more than 280,000 asymptomatic women—women who were not aware of a tumor in their breasts—more than 2,000 cancers were detected. Of these, 762 were in women under age 50 and 1,283 were in women over this age.

In this study, mammography was shown to be the single most effective way of detecting breast cancer. In the younger age group, mammography alone picked up the tumor in 36.4 percent of the cases; physical examination alone detected the tumor in only 13 percent. In the older-age women, mammography only detected a lesion in 42.1 percent as contrasted to 6.7 percent by physical examination only. These data clearly show that mammography is by far the single most effective way of detecting an early cancer of the breast.

It is important to know these facts because there has been some controversy over the use of mammography because of the associated radiation exposure. Theoretically, it would be desirable to avoid all forms of radiation; nevertheless, given the practical goal and beneficial results of detecting ever-earlier breast cancer, mammography is vitally important. The early furor about radiation exposure was probably overstated and further improvements in equipment have decreased the amount of radiation exposure in mammography. Thus, the medical consensus at present is that the risk of developing radiation-induced breast cancer from mammography, particularly in comparison to the benefits of this examination, is miniscule.

The level of undetected breast cancer in the United States is high. Approximately half a million American women have this disease and are unaware of it. Mammography clearly has demonstrated its ability to pick up early cancer of the breast at a stage when the cure rate can be considered excellent. Consequently, mammography is a vital and relatively risk-free technique for detecting earlier breast cancers.

Mammography should be used with circumspection in screening a younger asymptomatic women because of the relatively lower occurrence of breast cancer in this age population and the difficulty of detecting cancers in the denser breast tissue of the younger female.

Though mammography can make the difference between life and death in breast cancer and its judicious use is of great importance, it is not perfect; mammography has about an 85 percent accuracy rate in detecting cancer of the breast or in ruling it out. It is more effective in the post-menopausal female than in the pre-menopausal woman because of the denser nature of young breast tissue. This may be the reason Susan's mammogram did not detect her cancer. It also illustrates the veracity of the aphorism that a negative mammogram does not eliminate the necessity for biopsy of a tumor that is palpated in the breast.

Intra-Oral Cancer

Intra-oral cancer includes cancer of the lips, the tongue, the floor of the mouth, the buccal mucosa (the lining of the cheek), the gums or gingiva, the hard and soft palate (the roof of the mouth), and the pharynx (the area of the throat at the back of the mouth).

In the United States, 30,000 new cases of cancer developed in these tissues this year. More than twice as many men develop these cancers as did women and they are most frequent in males over the age of 40. More than 9,400 patients died of these cancers this year.

Deaths from intra-oral cancers are particularly distressing because most of these cancers are subject to early detection by inspection and palpation. The cure rate with early detection is excellent—in excess of 80 percent. However, the cure rate for advanced intra-oral cancer drops to about 15 percent. Furthermore, the type of death in this cancer is a dreadful experience. Advanced intra-oral cancer is accompanied by pain, disfigurement of the head and neck area, bleeding, discharge of mucus and saliva and marked impairment in the ability to swallow and speak. Breathing difficulty may also ensue. Worse, the victim is fully aware of his circumstances throughout this ordeal. Of all deaths from cancer, this is among the most harrowing. Early diagnosis, achieved by simple methods of detection, can often prevent this outcome.

As with other forms of cancer, there are certain groups at increased risk of developing this disease. Intra-oral cancers are found predominantly in those individuals who have a history of smoking and excess drinking. Cigarette smoking is usually involved, although individuals who smoke pipes and cigars also increase their chance of developing this tumor. Chewing tobacco and dipping snuff, which is a tobacco substance held in the cheek, have become major predisposing factors. People with these habits should give them up. If they don't, they should be particularly wary of the development of intra-oral tumors and should employ the self-detection techniques to be described. This is particularly vital since, presently, 60 percent of all oral cancers are well advanced by the time diagnosis is made.

Technique of Intra-Oral Examination

Examine your mouth monthly, using your birthdate as the day to do this important study. The examination can be done in front of the bathroom mirror with a good light illuminating the lips and interior of the mouth. Frequently, however, a light which is above the mirror will shine directly into your eyes, and not very effectively into your mouth, making inspection difficult. To remedy this, use a flashlight which can be directed into your mouth without the overhead light beaming into your eyes. This puts the illumination in your mouth where you want it, and provides a more effective way of performing the examination. Some people find a large hand-held mirror is better than a mirror fixed to a wall.

Remove any dentures prior to the exam. Inspect the outer surfaces of the lips. Then, with the fingers, pull down the lips. Examine their inner surfaces carefully (Fig. 2A). Then retract the cheeks with your fingers and inspect the gums and the inner surfaces of the cheeks (the buccal mucosa) (Fig. 2B). You may notice projecting from the surface of the buccal mucosa at about the level of the second upper molar tooth a small mound, or papilla, which is the site of the entrance of the parotid salivary duct into the mouth. Saliva may jet from this normal structure.

Next, open the mouth widely, protrude the tongue and inspect its surface, then retract the cheek to one side with the fingers and, with the tongue protruding as far as it can go to the opposite side, inspect carefully the lateral edges of the tongue and the floor of the mouth (Fig. 2C). Cancers of the tongue characteristically

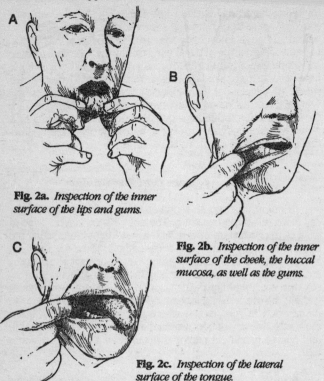

Fig. 2a. *Inspection of the inner surface of the lips and gums.*

Fig. 2b. *Inspection of the inner surface of the cheek, the buccal mucosa, as well as the gums.*

Fig. 2c. *Inspection of the lateral surface of the tongue.*

arise from the tongue's sides, or lateral surfaces and on its under-surface. They practically never arise on its top, or dorsum, so pay particular attention to the lateral aspects and undersurfaces of the tongue.

Then raise the tip of the tongue to the top of the mouth, or palate, and inspect its undersurfaces and the floor of the mouth (Fig 2D). On the undersurface of the tongue you will note two ridges of tissue running from front to back. In addition, in the floor of the mouth you will see the frenulum of the tongue, a sharp, thin fold of tissue running from the tongue to the floor of

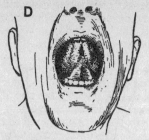

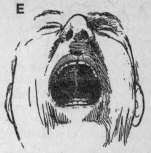

Fig. 2d. *Inspection of the undersurface of the tongue and floor of the mouth.*

Fig. 2e. *Inspection of the palate —the roof of the mouth.*

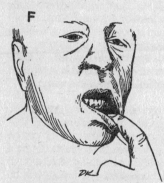

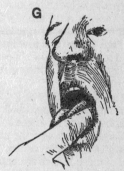

Fig. 2f. *Palpation of the lips and buccal mucosa.*

Fig. 2g. *Palpation of the tongue.*

the mouth in the midline. You will also notice in the floor of the mouth two prominent furrows which run from back to the front and middle of the mouth where they end in two prominent projections. These are the submaxillary ducts leading from the submaxillary glands below the jaw and which carry saliva into the mouth. All of these are perfectly normal structures.

When this phase has been completed, open the mouth widely, throw back the head and inspect the roof of the mouth (Fig. 2E). There you will see the hard and soft palate. Some persons have a congenital bony overgrowth in the middle of the hard palate

103

called a torus palatinus. This is a perfectly normal structure and is not a tumor. Finally, protrude the tongue, shine your flashlight into the back of the mouth, and say "Ahh." This will allow you to inspect the pharynx, or throat, at the back of the mouth.

When this has been done, use your finger to palpate all of the intra-oral tissues which you have just inspected. Bring your finger along the inner surfaces of the lip, (Fig 2F), the buccal mucosa, the tongue—especially along its sides and its undersurface (Fig. 2G), the floor of the mouth, the gums, the palate and then back into the pharynx. If the finger goes further posteriorly, you may gag.

What telltale signs are you looking for in this exam? The earliest evidence of cancer is a reddened area called erythroplasia, or erythema. Normally, most of the intra-oral tissues have a salmon-pink color and are thin and shiny and appear healthy. Erythroplasia is characterized by a magenta-red appearance of the tissues in any one area. The area of erythroplasia is velvety in consistency, compared to the thin, silky appearance of healthy intra-oral tissues. If you detect such a lesion, seek medical or dental attention.

You must also look for the presence of leukoplakia. As the name implies, leukoplakia consists of a dead, white plaque. This particular lesion has some substance or thickness to it and can be seen and also felt with the palpated finger. Leukoplakia can be a pre-malignant lesion or may be associated with a cancer though most of these lesions are benign. Some intra-oral lesions will be predominantly white with specklings or red or vice versa. These are an indication to seek professional help.

Though erythroplasia and leukoplakia may be the earliest manifestations of intra-oral cancer, as the cancer progresses, further changes will become visible. You may note a small fissure or crack in these tissues. As the tumor process continues, ulceration, or destruction of tissue will occur, and an ulcer will develop. As the cancer enlarges, it will produce a raised, cauliflower, or fleshy-looking, tumor. The classical appearance of moderately advanced cancer is that of central ulceration surrounded by an elevated peripheral tumor.

Palpation is an important part of the intra-oral examination and should be done on the tissues you have just inspected. The most important finding is that of induration, or thickening of tissue. Normally, intra-oral structures are smooth, soft, pliable and non-tender. An early cancer may manifest itself to the examining finger by an area of firmness or thickening. Later tumors reveal a mass which can be felt. If ulceration has occurred, tenderness may be present. If the tissues manifest friability or fragility to the gentle examining finger, or if bleeding occurs after such palpation, medical or dental attention should be sought.

In both inspection and palpation of the mouth, you have the benefit of bilaterality, i.e., you can compare one side of the mouth to the other. A significant change on one side should be readily detected when compared to the normal finding on the other.

It is very safe to say that if Todd had been performing a monthly examination like this, his outlook would have been appreciably improved. His cancer on the lateral border of the tongue should have been readily visible and palpable. He would not have missed this lesion because he could compare the two sides of the tongue, left and right, both by inspection and by palpation. This comparison would have clearly showed that the involved left side of the tongue had an area of ulceration, tenderness and thickening which was absent on the right. Knowing the significance of this finding, he would have come to his physician when the tumor was much smaller and the prognosis far better. Unfortunately, he knew nothing about the causes of cancer of the tongue, never examined himself prophylactically and ignored symptoms when they did develop.

There are many, too many, Todds in our country.

Salivary Gland Cancer

Cancer of the salivary glands is relatively uncommon. About 1,000 patients each year develop these cancers with a cure rate of 55 percent. As with other cancers, the cure rate could be improved with prompt diagnosis. Early detection is relatively easy to accomplish in the salivary glands because they are located immediately beneath the skin and are amenable to palpation and inspection.

The major salivary glands are the parotid, submaxillary and sublingual glands. The parotid gland is located in the face immediately in front of the ear (Fig. 3). It is the most common site

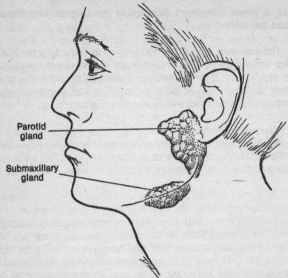

Fig. 3. *Locations of the parotid and submaxillary gland.*

of salivary gland cancer. Remembering this is the area which swells in mumps gives you a good idea of its location. Normally, the parotid glands extend to just under the lobule of the tip of the ear and cannot be felt.

The nerve which controls the muscles of facial expression runs through the parotid, and allows us to close our eyes, wrinkle our forehead and smile. Cancer of the parotid may invade this facial nerve, producing weakness or even paralysis of this structure. If this cancer develops, it may manifest itself by weakness in the facial muscles causing inability to retract the mouth, close the eye, etc.

Examination of the parotid should include both inspection and palpation. Look at the parotid area to see if a tumor is visible. Check for involvement of the facial nerve, which as noted, would be manifested by weakness of the facial muscles. Then palpate the parotid by pressing the tips of your fingers gently over this area in stroking and patting motions to detect any induration (hard-

106

ness) or tumor formation. Remember to compare one parotid against the other.

The submaxillary glands are located in the upper neck, just under the jawbone. Saliva is delivered to the mouth through a duct which you have previously seen during your intra-oral exam exiting in the midline of the floor of the mouth. If inspection or palpation in the area of the submaxillary gland reveals a tumor mass, professional assistance should be sought.

Sublingual gland cancers are extremely uncommon. They emerge as masses in the floor of the mouth, which can be detected by your intra-oral examination.

Thyroid Gland Cancer

Cancer of the thyroid develops in about 10,600 patients annually in the United States. Fortunately, these cancers are not very aggressive and claim only about 1100 deaths per year. Again, however, it is desirable to detect these lesions early. The thyroid gland is located in the root of the neck, just below and lateral to the larynx or voice box (Fig. 4).

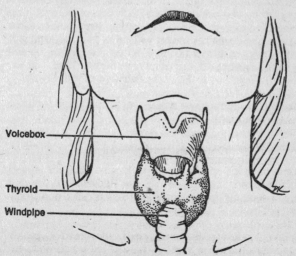

Voicebox

Thyroid

Windpipe

Fig. 4. *Location of the thyroid gland.*

A history of irradiation therapy is common in patients with thyroid cancer, particularly when irradiation therapy was administered in infancy or childhood. In the past, children were given radiation for such conditions as an enlarged thymus gland in the chest, infected and enlarged tonsils, ringworm and acne. This treatment was discontinued in this country about 1960. The risk of developing thyroid cancer appears to be directly proportional to the amount of radiation absorbed by the thyroid. Unfortunately, these tumors can develop up to 30 years after the radiation treatment.

Check for the presence of a possible thyroid tumor by inspecting the area in the front of the neck to either side of the voice box and the windpipe. Examine this area in the mirror. When you swallow, the thyroid gland may be observed to move up and down in the neck, particularly in slender-necked individuals. The size of the gland is similar on both sides. If a tumor is present in the thyroid, it may appear as an asymmetrical bulge which moves up and down in the front of the neck during this swallowing movement.

Next, palpate the thyroid gently for tumors (Fig. 5). In most cases, the normal thyroid gland cannot be felt. However, if a tumor is present, it may be palpable. Place the fingers of the right hand along the left neck in the butterfly area of the thyroid and swallow. Drinking a small amount of water will aid in your swallowing. If a tumor is present, it may be felt as a firm mass, riding up and down in the neck under the examining fingers. Then, use the fingers of the left hand to check the right lobe of your thyroid.

Encouragingly, the great majority of thyroid gland swellings are benign conditions.

Cancer in Lymph Nodes

Cancers which arise primarily in lymph nodes are termed lymphomas; lymphomas are divided into Hodgkin's disease, and a group of other malignant lymph node tumors called non-Hodgkin's lymphoma.

A lymph node may also be enlarged by the spread of a cancer from another organ. This was the cause of the lymph node enlargement in the left neck of Todd McCormick.

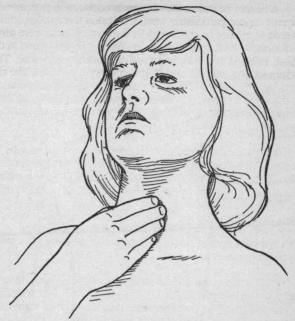

Fig. 5. *Palpation of the thyroid gland.*

It is recommended that you inspect and palpate your lymph nodes once a month. In the overwhelming majority of cases, any lymph node enlargement will be the result of a benign condition, such as an infection, and not cancer. You should check the lymph nodes in three areas: the neck, the axillae or armpits, and in the groin (Fig 6).

In the neck, the three most common sites for lymph node enlargement are the submandibular area, located just beneath and under the lower jawbone on either side. A second site is in the middle of the neck about three inches lateral to the voice box. The third site is the supra-clavicular area of the neck, located low in the neck just above the collarbone.

The axillary lymph nodes—those located in the armpits—should also be examined. This is best done by gently palpating

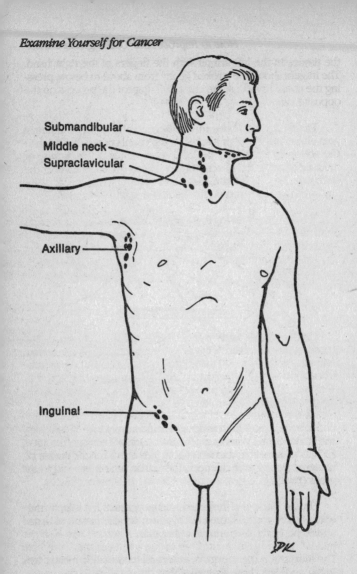

Fig. 6. *Location of major lymph node areas.*

the tissues in the left armpit with the fingers of the right hand. The fingers should be stroked gently from above to below, pressing the tissue in against the chest wall. Repeat the process on the opposite side.

Finally, lymph nodes may enlarge in the groin or inguinal area either just above or just below the connection of the thigh to the abdomen. This may be the site of either a lymphoma, or metastatic cancer from such primary organs as the genitalia or the skin of the leg. Once again, in the overwhelming majority of cases, any swelling which you do find in this area will be benign.

What are you looking for? Lymph nodes are normally present in all three of these areas—neck, axilla (armpit) or groin. You may be able to palpate them as firm, non-tender, pea or lima bean sized nodules. If the nodes are bigger than this, you should get a medical evaluation.

Cancer of the Testis

Cancer of the testis if a relatively uncommon tumor, but nevertheless more than 5,500 cases occur annually in the United States and more than 400 men die of this condition. There is little information as to why testicular cancer develops. However, it is seen more frequently in patients in whom the testis has not descended fully into the scrotum.

Although testicular cancer is comparatively rare, it is nonetheless the most common cancer in U.S. males between the ages of 15 and 34 years, accounting for 19 percent of cancer deaths in this age group. The incidence of testicular cancer in whites has risen in recent decades; the tumor is rare in American blacks.

The symptoms of testicular cancer include a lump in the testis, a swollen or enlarged testis, pain, and a sensation of heaviness or dragging in the groin or scrotum.

Unlike most other organs, almost all tumors in the testis are cancer. However, also located within the scrotum is the epididymis—the duct from the testis—which can be the site of inflammation and can somewhat mimic the appearance of a testicular

111

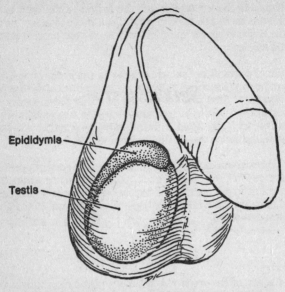

Fig. 7. *Location of testis and epididymis in scrotum.*

tumor (Fig. 7). Only a physician can distinguish between an enlargement of the testis, which is likely cancer, and enlargement of the epididymis, which is usually benign.

Monthly palpation of the testis, preferably during a hot shower, for the presence of a tumor is a useful process. A tumor manifests itself by an increase in size, firmness or weight of the testis. Any change in the testicular area is a cause for prompt medical evaluation.

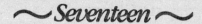

~Seventeen~

The Psychology of Cancer Detection

Certainly, there are many, many unanswered questions about cancer. One of the most complex is also the most basic: Why and how is the genetic material of a normal cell changed into genes coding for cancer? Current research suggests the existence of an oncogene residing within normal cells which can be "switched on" to induce cancer.

The ultimate answer to this biologic problem is obscure, but it is certainly no more obscure than understanding why certain people adopt and adhere to cancer-producing patterns of living and then ignore the signs and symptoms of cancer when they develop.

Unfortunately, clinicians frequently see individuals who ignore symptoms of cancer, coming for treatment only after periods of delay which allow dangerous—and perhaps fatal—growth of the tumor. We will probably unravel the biologic enigmas of cancer cell development long before the psychologic mechanisms of patient delay are fully fathomed.

Undoubtedly, there are a number of causes for this delay, including misinformation or lack of knowledge about cancer. Even in these days of widespread educational efforts, some people are still ignorant about cancer's symptoms. Quite simply, we must continue to improve our efforts to educate this group of our fellow citizens.

More difficult to understand and to help is the person who is aware of the early manifestations of cancer but who refuses to take action to help himself. Often, the cause of this inaction is fear and denial of the situation. Certainly, this is an understandable reaction; however, with the realization that early detection of many cancers is accompanied by excellent cure rates, fewer people will delay treatment because of anxiety.

Economic worries may precipitate delays, too. An individual may become aware of symptoms that suggest cancer but, because of the cost of medical help, defer seeking medical assistance. This should never be a cause for procrastination. Physicians will, and do, offer services without charge, or will adjust fees when circumstances warrant. Furthermore, there are free clinics in all areas of this country where appropriate care can be found. Though the setting for these clinics may lack frills, the care of the patient will be of high quality.

A number of individuals will defer seeking medical attention because they want to do something else which they consider more important. These priorities may include immersing themselves in their careers or jobs. To a certain extent, this is understandable because making a livelihood is vital to all of us. However, health is more important than any job. Often these concerns about the job are only an excuse to defer medical attention, rather than a real fear of being fired or demoted. Remember: You can always find another job but you can't replace your health once it is gone.

Much more difficult to understand are people who consider social functions, recreational activities and cultural pursuits more important than the need for medical evaluation. It is not at all uncommon to find people who will defer a cancer check-up or treatment for a number of months because they wish to take a vacation. These misguided choices can have fatal results. The question here is simple enough. What are your priorities?

So, what attitude should you have toward cancer? You should have a prudent, appropriate concern for your health based on awareness of the nature of cancer. If you suspect you have a tumor, you should neither panic nor bury your head in the sand. Don't give way to a feeling of fatalism, which in most circumstances is unwarranted. Knowledge, emotional maturity and the ability to react rationally to a possible health threat are the keystones to taking the prudent actions which may save your life.

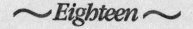

~ Eighteen ~

Warning Signs

The American Cancer Society has performed a valuable service by identifying seven warning signs of cancer. These signs are:

- Change in bowel or bladder habits
- A sore that does not heal
- Unusual bleeding or discharge
- Thickening or lump in breast or elsewhere
- Indigestion or difficulty in swallowing
- Obvious change in wart or mole
- Nagging cough or hoarseness

If you have one of these symptoms, you should report to your physician or clinic promptly because they could—repeat, *could*—indicate cancer. All too often, these warning signs are ignored with unpleasant consequences.

Be reassured by the fact that the overwhelming majority of people who have one or more of these signs do not have cancer. The symptom or physical change was caused by some other disease process. Nevertheless, the cause for these changes can only be determined by medical evaluation. If you have one or more of these warning signs, make sure you get this evaluation promptly!

Susan Webster was aware of the significance of a mass in the breast because her mother had breast cancer, and also from her reading on the subject. Her prompt response led to quick medical attention and the interval between her first symptom and diagnosis was only a few days. In contrast, Todd McCormick paid little heed to the pain in his mouth and jaw, and a number of months went by before he sought professional help.

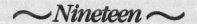

~Nineteen~

"Yes, You Do Have Cancer..."

Your Reaction

These are fateful—but not necessarily fatal—words. Almost half of those who hear these stunning, frightening words will survive. Nevertheless, this message comes with numbing surprise. When the initial shock has worn off, the next typical reaction is one of disbelief—that this cannot be happening to you. This phase often evolves to a "Why me?" feeling. All of the phases are understandable and normal. Be consoled by one fact, however; at this moment, you are at your absolute psychological low. From this point, almost invariably, your emotional status will improve. Once you are sure of the diagnosis, uncertainty is eliminated and you will soon react in a more positive manner.

Your emotional responses are very important because they

play a major role in your ability to select a treatment program. Stay cool, so that your decision-making processes will function well. Accept this situation and *attack* your problem. Most of the time, your prognosis is not as black as you may think.

First, be assured that you can handle the situation. Hundreds of thousands of others have done so successfully; you can also, and you will. Have confidence in yourself, even in the face of this greatest psychological test of your life. Take it one day at a time. It will all work itself out.

A frank and open relationship with your physician is of paramount importance. He should be telling you all he knows about your condition and you should be asking him any questions you have in mind. This candid exchange of information is very important in establishing a solid and reassuring relationship between the two of you; such a relationship will be of great support to you in the days ahead. If you feel that this open communication is not present, express this concern to your physician. Discussing your perception with your doctor should clear the air and establish the supportive dialogue you need. Upon occasion, human personalities being what they are, you may not be able to relate easily to your individual physician. If this is the case, explain this to him and seek medical care with someone else.

The Importance of Your Decisions

Your first cancer treatment is of critical importance, because if this first treatment fails and the tumor recurs, the success of secondary treatment is not as good. Your first chance is your best chance for a cure. This principal holds true whether the first treatment effort is surgery, irradiation therapy or chemotherapy. It is of utmost importance, therefore, that competent physicians plan your initial treatment and implement it with appropriate aggressiveness.

You can do nothing to alter the inhererent biological properties of your cancer, but you *can* control these treatment choices, which are of such great importance. The stakes are too high to scrimp on time, effort or cost. Though cancer is an implacable foe, it can be overcome. To do this, however, you must get the best treatment available.

Becoming Informed

The more you know about all aspects of your cancer, the better your decisions will be. *Now* is the time to acquire the information upon which you will base these decisions.

First, you need to know about your disease. Precisely, what type of cancer do you have? In what organ is it located? Has the disease spread? What types of treatment are available to you? What is your prognosis? Understanding your disease is a vital process in deciding what to do about it. Learn as much as you can.

Realize, however, there is a limit to the amount of information that you should seek to acquire. It is impossible to take a crash course in oncology under these circumstances. Delving too deeply into highly technical works on cancer is probably more counterproductive than helpful. Attempting to weigh the results of reports in the medical literature, which are often confusing and conflicting, can cause anxiety in the most resolute of hearts. Generally, then, you will have acquired adequate information when you understand those principals of the disease which will have an effect on your treatment choices.

A more important subject for you to research is where you can get the best medical care. You must identify qualified oncologists, determine the location of specialized resources such as irradiation therapy equipment and the availability of multi-disciplinary cancer consultation services. Familiarize yourself with the possibilities of treatment both in your community and at more distant locations.

Sources of Information

You can get this information from a number of sources:

- The National Cancer Institute has established a Cancer Information Service (CIS) in a number of regions about the country. You may call the CIS toll-free at 1-800-525-3777. Trained personnel will answer your questions and will supply the information which you need about treatment facilities (see appendix).
- The American Cancer Society has local chapters throughout

the United States which offer a host of supportive services for the cancer patient. Among these are an information program which will inform you about the patient care opportunities available to you (see appendix).

• Comprehensive Cancer Centers are institutions which have been recognized by the National Cancer Institute as having major oncologic programs. These centers can offer information about your treatment possibilities (see appendix).

• Medical schools in your vicinity will also have recommendations concerning qualified physicians and facilities. Many of these will be available in the medical school itself.

• The medical society in your community will usually have a list of physicians who specialize in oncology. This can be a valuable source of information for you.

• Your physician, if he is not an oncologist himself, will be aware of individuals in your community who have special oncologic training. Furthermore, your doctor should suggest a physician or physicians who will be most suited to your medical needs and your personality requirements.

• The P.D.Q. System is a computer data base for the retrieval of cancer treatment information. It is operated by the National Cancer Institute in Bethesda, Maryland. The P.D.Q. data base contains short summaries on state-of-the-art treatment of specific cancers. It also describes hundreds of cancer therapy research protocols, including the objective of individual treatment programs and patient entry criteria. It lists institutions where treatment programs are under investigation and names a contact person at each institution who can provide more information.

*Importantly, the P.D.Q. System lists the names of oncologists who are members of recognized oncology organizations. The P.D.Q. System can list the names of these oncologists and their specialties, e.g. surgical oncology, medical oncology, etc. by specific cities in the United States. Your physician can use the P.D.Q. to identify these specialists in your locality.

*The P.D.Q. System is accessible through the National Library of Medicine's computer system. Presently, 3,000 MEDLARS (Medical Literature Abstracting and Retrieval Service) Centers in the United States have such access. These MEDLARS units are typically located in medical schools and major hospitals. Searches of the data base can be submitted by physicians at any of these locations.

*In addition to MEDLARS, commercial data base vendors make this material available to physician subscribers. These vendors are the BRS/Saunders' System, Colleague and the MEDIS System of Mead Data Central. In addition, a third vendor will be licensed in Europe—Fondation Suisse Telmed.

*Finally, individual physicians with personal computers can obtain access to the data base by obtaining their own access code.

*Utilization of the P.D.Q. will give up-to-the-minute information on the lastest advances in cancer treatment and the most recent lists of cancer specialists by locality. The data base is being constantly updated and expanded.

Making Your Choice

The diagnosis is established; you have cancer. Now what?

First of all, be reassured that you have adequate time to plan and initiate your counterattack. Remember it takes some cancers years to grow from one cell to one-half inch. So, a few days spent while you are mobilizing your resources against the cancer will not adversely impact your chances. There is enough time for you to obtain a second opinion about your condition. You should, however, not delay in obtaining these consultative opinions.

Most importantly, don't be panicked into almost immediate treatment. For many tumors, e.g. breast, skin, colon, stomach etc., a biopsy may be obtainable prior to treatment. Be wary of the advice that a definitive surgical procedure must be performed at the same time, or within a day or so of the return of a positive biopsy. In some cases immediate surgery may be necessary, but usually after the biopsy there is time for treatment planning.

Conversely, you must avoid the danger of deferring your decisions for a prolonged period while you obtain repeated consultations. Prolonged "shopping" for an opinion which you want to hear is counterproductive. There is a delicate balance between the time needed for getting all the reasonable information you need and an inordinate delay in decision making which is caused by wishful thinking or by your inability to come to a conclusion. Proceed carefully and promptly in this very important phase of your campaign against cancer.

"Yes, You Do Have Cancer ..."

Make the decision which is best for you, weighing a host of factors, including the obvious ones of the nature and extent of your tumor and the complexity of its treatment. Other considerations include your personal psychological reactions to the different settings where your treatment may be procured. There is no one "best" place for treatment of your cancer. In fact, you are probably located near a number of facilities where you can obtain superior care. Generally, however, there are two settings in which you may obtain proper oncologic attention—cancer centers and local medical facilities. These settings will be discussed separately.

Cancer Centers

Approximately 150 cancer centers are scattered throughout the United States. Some centers are concerned only with basic research and do not provide patient care. Others are predominantly clinical in their activities.

The Comprehensive Cancer Centers are, in general, the largest of these centers. The designation of Comprehensive Cancer Center is made by the federal government's National Cancer Institute only after a rigorous review of the center's activites which must include high-quality programs in clinical and basic research, in patient care activities and in cancer control. (See appendix for list of these comprehensive cancer centers and other centers). Typically, these centers are connected with large universities.

If you opt for treatment in a cancer center, you may safely assume that you'll be receiving the highest quality care. Appointment to the medical staff of such a center is quite competitive and almost invariably the personnel who will be caring for you have demonstrated high levels of competence in their specialties. Additionally, they will be aware of the latest developments in cancer research in institutions all around the world.

Many, although not all, of the patients who are treated in cancer centers are on research protocols. This means that new techniques or drugs are being used in an effort to combat the cancer. You do not have to participate in an investigational study to be treated in these centers, nor will you be urged to do so. However, this option is open to you.

124

There are advantages to being on a protocol study. You receive the best treatment known to acknowledged experts in cancer; you enjoy meticulous patient care, and you are evaluated more frequently and tested more extensively than patients who are not on protocol, because your physicians are interested in acquiring as much data as possible about the efficacy of the treatment being offered. This does entail some inconveniences to you, but also assures meticulous and detailed evaluation of your progress. Protocol research advances knowledge about cancer and has produced dramatic improvement in many cancer situations.

One negative aspect of treatment as a cancer center may be location. The center may be at a distance from your home, making travel inconvenient, disruptive to your family, and expensive. Also, for some people who have not been away from home very much, this dislocation may be upsetting.

Community Care

If you opt for care in your own community, be assured it is possible to receive superior medical attention in this setting. Large numbers of oncologists in practice in community settings have had the benefit of excellent training in cancer centers. The majority of these oncologists are medical oncologists or chemotherapists. Less numerous than the medical oncologists, but also well trained and specializing in malignant disease, are surgical, radiation, gynecologic and pediatric oncologists. These specialists have pursued additional training in cancer after completing the requirements for their specialty boards in, for example, surgery, and obstetrics and gynecology. It is recommended that you have an oncologist from one of these specialty areas either in charge of your case or playing an important role in decision-making. It is further recommended you have one physician, usually an oncologist, coordinating the treatment efforts.

The question is often asked—how can you determine the competence of an individual physician. Unfortunately, you can't. However, you can get a good feeling for his standing among his peers by appropriate inquiry. If you are seeking an oncologist, find out if he has passed his specialty boards. You can also determine if he is a member of one of the major oncologic associations

125

in this country. Admission to these organizations comes only after stringent peer review. Ask your family physician to recommend an oncologist.

Unfortunately, some people don't want to take advice. They ask for a recommendation for a competent specialist and, when provided a list of such names, they opt for someone else. Please...if you ask for advice from someone who should know, evaluate their recommendations carefully.

Almost as important as your choice of a physician will be your choice of the hospital where your treatment will be performed. Physicians have a limited number of hospitals with which they are affiliated, a factor which must be considered by you. You may have to decide to use a different doctor or hospital, if one is not affiliated with the other.

Your choice of a hospital for treatment will play an important role in the success of your care. Consequently, it is important for you to know which hospitals are committed to quality cancer-patient care. The American College of Surgeons has performed an impressive and valuable service in reviewing and analyzing the credentials of hospital cancer programs. The Commission on Cancer of the College has established criteria which a hospital must meet to have an approved program. These criteria include the existence of a multi-disciplinary committee on the hospital staff which reviews cancer activites. Educational conferences and tumor boards must be held frequently to ensure that physicians on the staff have access to the latest information on cancer and to multi-disciplinary consultation. Finally, a cancer registry must be in operation listing all cancer patients who are treated by the institution by diagnosis. The registry follows these patients to determine their survival rates. Additionally, cancer registries perform frequent analyses of patients survival experience for the hospital.

You are well advised to take into consideration these designations by the College of Surgeons in selecting your hospital (See appendix). Acceptance in these programs indicates that high standards of organization, personnel selection and review are being undertaken. This is not to suggest, however, that high quality programs do not exist in hospitals which have not applied for approval by the College.

Regardless of the treatment setting which you choose, have the microscopic pathology slides read by another pathologist. Occasionally, there may be disagreement in diagnosis which might be of considerable importance. This does not happen very often, but it does happen.

Again, before beginning treatment, all options should be explained to you by your physician team. You should have a multi-disciplinary approach to patient care. In a hospital approved by the College of Surgeons, you may ask to have your case presented to the local tumor board for discussion by cancer specialists from a number of disciplines. Such discussions cannot help but aid your treatment program.

Inquire if any of the treatment facilities in your commuunity are associated with a comprehensive cancer center or with one of the cooperative cancer research groups. With either of these associations, you know that oncologists in your community are collaborating with leading oncologists nationwide in research studies indicating that high-quality care is available.

Finally, regardless of the treatment setting, you may be forced to make choices between alternative forms of therapy. For example, you may have to select between surgery or irradiation therapy for cancer of the breast, or between irradiation therapy and chemotherapy for lymphoma. Admittedly, such choices are perplexing, confusing and they produce anxiety. Nevertheless, although these choices are difficult, be reassured that in the long term either of the proposed therapies will probably yield approximately equivalent results. If they did not achieve essentially similar success rates, one or the other would have been dropped as a treatment option. Therefore, the choice is mainly one of personal preference based on your individual interest and characteristics, rather than on the relative merits of treatment successes.

One particularly distressing situation—for patient and physician alike—is the search for a "miracle cure" by a patient who cannot accept the reality of his disease situation and finds no solace in the treatment options which are offered. Even intelligent people fall prey to this situation and will initiate an extensive, expensive and debilitating search for a quick miracle cure that simply does not exist. Oncologists are aware of all treatment options. Unfortunately, there are at present no miracle drugs or treatments that will quickly and dramatically cure you. Patients expend their physical, emotional and financial resources in a fruitless quest for something that simply does not exist. Under the trying circumstances of a cancer diagnosis, patients and their families may turn to quacks for medical care. Please stay away from the charlatan.

Follow-Up

A very important aspect of your total battle against cancer is follow-up care. Once you have had a significant form of cancer you should be checked periodically for life to assure that you stay in excellent health. These periodic check-ups assure you that if any recurrence of the disease does manifest itself, it will be detected at the earliest possible moment when a chance for a cure or for prolonged control of the cancer may still exist. Also, a patient who has had one cancer is at elevated risk of developing other cancers. For example, the woman who has had a breast cancer does have an increased chance, in comparison to the general population, of acquiring cancer in the opposite breast.

Follow-up evaluation will give you the maximal chance of permanent control of your cancer. After the initial anxiety of returning for the first check-up abates, these examinations will pay big emotional dividends because they will confirm that you are in excellent health.

Change Your Pattern of Living

You detected your cancer early in its development; you went for medical assistance to skilled and competent physicians. The disease has been erradicated. You have conscientiously embarked on a periodic follow-up program with your physician or oncologist. All of these steps help assure you of a healthy life.

However, there is one final requirement to further improve your odds against cancer. This time we must improve your odds against the development of a new, or second, cancer which may arise in the same organ as the original tumor, or in a closely-related structure. The second cancer may be caused by the same factor or factors that precipitated the first. For example, if you have had successful treatment for a cancer of the tongue and had been a smoker, you *must* stop your smoking promptly. If you do not, you may develop a second cancer in the intra-oral tissues or in the lung.

Unfortunately, it is not uncommon to see a successfully-treated cancer patient who, after a number of years, succumbs to a second cancer produced by the same causative factors. Nothing is more tragic. You have worked hard to beat cancer the first time around. Don't push your luck with a second cancer. Instead, change your pattern of living to a healthy one.

~ *Twenty* ~

You, in Society

Until now, we have concentrated solely on you as an individual—on ways in which you can prevent the occurrence of cancer, or can detect this disease at the earliest possible moment if it does develop. However, there are other steps you can take to improve cancer cure rates. You, as an individual, must participate in the struggle against this grim disease with your fellow citizens.

In the early 1970's, the American people, through their Congress, committed themselves to a national program to eliminate or control cancer. This mandate was enacted into law by the Congress and, as a result, federal support for cancer research, education and treatment was abundant in that decade. Thankfully, this support has stimulated unprecedented discoveries in the realm of biology. The cure rate for cancer has been improving steadily, if slowly, and there is optimism for the future. Cancer was—and remains—the primary health concern of the American people; unfortunately, the commitment to the program against cancer has begun to waiver in certain sectors of the federal government. It would be tragic indeed if support for cancer research were to decrease at this time when there is real promise of substantial improvement in the future. You and your fellow citizens must insist that the federal government continue its support of the struggle against cancer. Inform your elected officials in both the executive and legislative branches of your support for adequate cancer research funding.

A second way which you can manifest your commitment to this cause is to support the organizations and activities which are furthering the war against cancer.

The American Cancer Society is a national volunteer organization which for many decades has spearheaded the drive against this disease. The Society, through its individual chapters, had made outstanding contributions in supporting cancer research and patient care. Research discoveries, made possible through Society support, have been of inestimable value in advancing the cure rates against this condition. In addition, the Society has supported patient care activities and has undertaken a wide-spread program in education, in both professional and public spheres. The American Cancer Society has done an extremely commendable job and is worthy of your support.

If you wish to become more directly involved in the war against cancer, you may contribute your personal efforts or your fiscal support to any of the cancer research centers located around the country. These institutions welcome volunteer help for any of a number of programs. They also need your financial assistance. Cancer research is an expensive proposition.

Finally, because there is widespread public awareness of cancer-producing factors in our society—such as tobacco and alcohol—society should take steps to eliminate or minimize these factors. The classic example of the need for such societal action lies in the tobacco industry. Tobacco is a major health hazard and every effort must be made to control its use. It is obvious, however, that legislation which attempts to stifle the individual's right to make a decision is counterproductive. For example, an attempt to ban the sale of cigarettes would be ludicrous. Equally ludicrous, however, is the use of your tax dollars to support tobacco growing.

In the process of discouraging tobacco production however, the personal and financial plight of the tobacco farmer must be kept in mind. If federal subsidies are removed, ways must be found to assist this farmer in seeking other agricultural endeavors.

As another example, you and society must take further and more effective steps in establishing more healthful patterns of alcohol consumption. Once again, the attempt to ban drinking is impossible. Nevertheless, efforts must be made to have all of us— especially our teenagers—aware of the devastating toll which alcohol inflicts. Our society has been far too passive in this regard and excessive alcohol use has been quietly condoned. This is a major—and costly—mistake.

～ *Twenty-One* ～

The Bottom Line

Cancer, in many of its forms, is a controllable and curable disease. There has been a steady and dramatic improvement in cure rates: in the 1920s, the cure rate for cancer was only about 20 percent; in the 1950s, about one patient in three was cured; now, the cure rate has reached about 50 percent. This dramatic improvement has not come about by chance. This progress has been achieved as a result of vast research efforts in both the laboratory and in the clinic.

Only a few decades ago, all children who developed acute leukemia died of the disease, and 90 percent of them died within one year. An intensive research effort was launched to correct this terrible situation. New anti-cancer drugs were developed and their most effective utilization was studied intensively. The importance of antibiotic treatment for the infection which commonly arose in these disease-ravaged young patients was discovered. The contribution of X-ray treatment of the brain and the spinal cord to eliminate leukemic cells became understood. The critical importance of minimizing exposure to infectious organisms in the environment was appreciated and methods to secure such isolation were achieved. The importance of the psychological and social support of the patient and family became recognized.

Each of these advances was achieved by a series of slow, painstaking and often heart-rending steps. They were made possible only by the dedication of the young patients, their families, their attending physicians and supporting scientists. The courage of the young patients was the indispensable factor in this epochal struggle. The cure rate of 50 percent which has been achieved for leukemic children is a testimony to the success of these struggles. The fact that half of them still die demands our commitment for the future. Such commitment will be successful against all cancers. With this dedication, the fear of cancer will be eliminated by the year 2000.

∼ *Twenty-Two* ∼

Follow-up Notes

On a routine follow-up visit, about five months after Todd McCormick's operation, an ulceration was noted in the floor of the mouth in the vicinity of the original cancer. At this same time, some thickening of the tissues in the left neck also became apparent. His doctors were uncertain whether these changes represented recurrent cancer or were caused by his previous surgical and irradiation treatments. After a period of observation of three weeks, the ulceration in the mouth was biopsied and revealed recurrent squamous cell cancer.

Having failed both surgical and radiation therapy treatment, Todd was referred to medical oncologists for consideration of chemotherapy. Although the chances of any substantial salvage were dim, chemotherapy was begun. However, impressive shrinkage of the tumor was noted and, at the end of his third month of treatment—which was performed on an outpatient basis—no residual cancer was noted. Todd returned to work in a satisfactory state of health.

Not long afterward, however, ulceration caused by the cancer again returned and, from this point on, progressed inexorably. Pain, which had disappeared after the operation, returned and increased steadily. The successive use of aspirin, codeine and opiates in progressively higher doses was necessary to keep Todd pain-free. The tumor mass in the left neck ulcerated through the skin and created a tract between the inside of the mouth and the skin, through which pus and saliva drained. Upon occasion, small episodes of bleeding occurred.

Todd remained at home, at his own request, during this time. However, substantial nursing and psychological problems developed which required readmission to the hospital because Mrs. McCormick, despite her dedicated efforts, was unable to cope with all of his needs. Todd began to experience difficulty in breathing due to obstruction by the tumor, especially when lying down. This caused him great distress. Consequently, a tracheostomy was performed under local anesthesia. This alleviated his air hunger and its concomitant anxiety. Chemotherapy had been stopped and the family met with his physician and social workers to determine the best means of palliation for him. Admission to a hospice was being planned when he developed a massive hemorrage in the open wound in the left neck and bled to death within a few minutes. He died approximately 11 months after seeing his doctor for the first time.

Final Autopsy Diagnosis

Name: McCormick, Todd H.
Age: 58
Sex: Male
Race: White
Pathology Number: 87A160
Hours Postmortem: ..13
Restrictions to Autopsy Examination: ..None
Unit Number: 733-14-24
Department: Surgery
Attending Physician: ..Patrick X. Ruggles, M.D.

Autopsy Performed By: ..Claudia A. Levy, M.D.

Admitted: ..7/26/87 at 10:05 a.m.

Died: ..8/13/87 at 8:45 p.m.

Date of Autopsy: ..8/14/87 at 9:45 a.m.

Requestor: Mrs. Todd McCormick (wife)

Clinical Summary: This 58-year-old white male had a commando type operation for squamous cell carcinoma metastatic to the left neck. Post-operatively, he was treated with radiation therapy totalling 6,000 rads to the left neck and intra-oral tissues. Biopsy proven recurrence was demonstrated and he was begun on chemotherapy. After initial response, tumor recurred in the mouth and in neck. He died of a massive hemmorage from the neck.

Gross Autopsy Findings: The body is that of an emaciated white male measuring 163 centimeters. Weight is approximately 65 kg. A tracheostomy has recently been performed and a Shiley tracheostomy tube in place. There is a large fungating tumor in the left upper neck which has produced extensive ulceration. A fistulous tract is present into the oropharynx. Blood clot is present intra-orally and in the ulcerated wound. On removal of this clot, a rupture of the common carotid artery is visible. Upon opening the pleural cavities, multiple nodules are visible throughout both lungs, compatible with metastatic disease. Large mediastinal nodes are visible, compatible with metastatic cancer. The heart and pericardial sac are essentially normal. The abdominal cavity was opened and revealed . . .

Final Autopsy Diagnosis:

1) Squamous cell carcinoma of the tongue, metastatic to the neck.
2) Ulceration of left neck tissues secondary to carcinoma.
3) Rupture of common carotid artery.
4) Metastatic squamous cell carcinoma to the lung.
5) Metastatic squamous cell carcinoma to liver.

****

Susan Webster saw her surgeon every two months during her first postoperative year. On none of these visits did she have any symptoms to report, nor was there any evidence of recurrent cancer. On each visit, a blood test, called a C.E.A., was performed to see if there was laboratory evidence of metastatic cancer. All of these blood tests were within normal limits. Periodic chest X-ray examinations and mammography also showed no abnormality.

In the second year after her operation, Susan was seen every three months. She continued in good health. At about this time she met, through her professional relationships, an attorney in whom she became interested. This interest, during the next several months, progressed to friendship and mutual regard, and then to love.

Susan was quite straightforward in telling him about her breast cancer and the operation. This made no difference at all to him because, as he said, he had fallen in love with Susan and not with her breasts. After a brief courtship, they were married.

About a year-and-a-half after her marriage, Susan decided to have reconstruction of the left breast performed. She did this primarily to avoid the nuisance of having to wear a prosthesis in her bra and also to facilitate her choice of clothes. This operation, which was performed by a plastic surgeon, produced a breast which was normal in size, contour and consistency. A nipple complex was created which was almost indistinguishable from the opposite normal nipple. The only indications of the previous mastectomy were a few scars in the breast area. Both Susan and her husband were very pleased with the results of the reconstruction.

In the five-and-a-half years since her mastectomy, Susan has continued to do well. There has been no evidence of recurrence of her cancer. Her followup visits now occur only twice a year. She has been promoted to a supervisory position in her accouting firm. Her husband has been a warm, supportive and communicative person. They love each other deeply. They share and enjoy a variety of professional, social, athletic and recreational activities. With their combined financial resources, they have purchased a very attractive home to which neither could have aspired independently. Susan's life is a full and happy one. She has almost forgotten that she ever had cancer.

THE END

～Suggested Diet Plans～

You can have a healthy diet by selecting foods from the Basic Four Food Guide for Meal Planning.

●MILK: 2 servings/adults
4 servings/teenagers
3 servings/children
8 oz. equals 1 serving.

Use skim or 1% milk, low fat cottage cheese, cheeses and yogurt.

●MEAT: 2 servings
FISH:
POULTRY:

1 oz. equals 1 serving.

Use poultry such as chicken, turkey and Cornish hen without skin, fish, dried beans and peas as meat substitutes. Limit beef, veal, pork and lamb to 3 or 4 servings per week. But, only lean cuts of meat.

●BREADS & STARCHES: 4 servings 1/2 C. pasta, cereal, potatoes; 1 slice bread equals 1 serving.

Use whole grain, fortified or enriched products such as cereals, breads and flours.

●FRUITS & VEGETABLES: 4 servings 1/2 C. cooked vegetables and fruits. 1/2 C. raw vegetables and fruits.

Use citrus fruits and juices daily as a source of vitamin C; green, leafy, and deep yellow vegetables as a source of vitamin A.

Remember to include a variety of foods in your diet each day. Drink 6 to 8 glasses of water. It is important to regulate your intake of fat to no more than 30 percent of the calories per day. The following sample meal plan provides a balanced diet containing approximately 1,600 calories with a caloric distribution of 52 percent carbohydrate, 20 percent protein and 28 percent fat.

Suggested Diet Plans

SAMPLE MENU	PORTION SIZE
Breakfast	
Sliced Strawberries, fresh	1 ¼ Cup
Unsweetened Orange Juice	½ Cup
Bran Flakes	¾ Cup
Whole Wheat Toast	1 slice
Margarine	1 teaspoon
Skim Milk	1 8oz. Cup
Lunch	
Sliced Turkey	2 ounces
on Whole Grain Bread	2 slices
Sliced Tomato on Romaine	3 slices
Lettuce	
Cantaloupe	1 Cup
Mayonnaise	1 Tablespoon
Skim Milk	1 8 oz. Cup
Dinner	
Fresh Flounder with	3 ounces
Mustard Sauce	
Wild Rice Pilaf	1 Cup
Broccoli Spears	2 stalks
Tossed Salad	1 Cup
Lemon Dressing	2 Tablespoons
Fresh Peach and Kiwi Dessert	1 medium, 1 large
Dinner Roll	1 small
Margarine	1 teaspoon

～Appendix 1～

Cancer Information Service

For information about cancer, call the Cancer Information Service toll-free number listed below for your state. In states not listed, call 800-638-6694. These services are funded by the federal government's National Cancer Institute.

Alabama: 1-800-292-6201

Alaska: 1-800-638-6070

California:
From Area Codes (213), (714)
and (805): 1-800-252-9066

Connecticut: 1-800-922-0824

Delaware: 1-800-523-3586

Florida: 1-800-432-5953

Georgia: 1-800-327-7332

Hawaii:
Oahu: 524-1234
Neighbor Islands: Ask operator
for Enterprise 6702

Illinois: 1-800-972-0586

Kentucky: 1-800-432-9321

Maine: 1-800-225-7034

Maryland: 1-800-492-1444

Massachusetts: 1-800-952-7420

Minnesota: 1-800-582-5262

New Hampshire: 1-800-225-7034

New Jersey:
(Northern) 1-800-223-1000
(Southern) 1-800-523-3586

New York State: 1-800-462-7255

New York City: (212) 794-7982

North Carolina: 1-800-672-0943

North Dakota: 1-800-328-5188

Appendix 1

Ohio: 1-800-282-6522

Pennsylvania: 1-800-822-3963

South Dakota: 1-800-328-5188

Texas: 1-800-392-2040

Vermont: 1-800-225-7034

Washington: 1-800-552-7212

Wisconsin: 1-800-362-8038

Comprehensive Cancer Centers

The institutions listed have been recognized as Comprehensive Cancer Centers by the National Cancer Institute. These centers have met rigorous criteria imposed by the National Cancer Advisory Board. They receive financial support from the National Cancer Institute, the American Cancer Society and many other sources.

ALABAMA
University of Alabama in Birmingham
  Comprehensive Cancer Center
Lurleen Wallace Tumor Institute
1824 6th Avenue South
Birmingham, Alabama 35294
Phone: (205) 934-5077

CALIFORNIA
University of Southern California
  Comprehensive Cancer Center
1441 Eastlake Avenue
Los Angeles, California 90033-0804
Phone: (213) 224-6416

UCLA-Jonsson Comprehensive Cancer Center
Louis Factor Health Sciences Bldg.
10833 LeConte Avenue
Los Angeles, California 90024
Phone: (213) 825-5268

CONNECTICUT
Yale Comprehensive Cancer Center
Yale University School of Medicine
333 Cedar Street
New Haven, Connecticut 06510
Phone: (203) 785-4095

DISTRICT OF COLUMBIA
Vincent T. Lombardi Cancer Research
  Center
Georgetown University Medical Center

3800 Reservoir Road, N.W.
Washington, D.C. 20007
Phone: (202) 625-7721

Howard University Cancer Research
  Center
College of Medicine
Department of Oncology
2041 Georgia Avenue, N.W.
Washington, D.C. 20060
Phone: (202) 636-7697

FLORIDA
Comprehensive Cancer Center for
  the State of Florida
University of Miami School of
  Medicine
1475 N.W. 12th Avenue
Miami, Florida 33101
Phone: (305) 545-7707

ILLINOIS
Illinois Cancer Council
36 South Wabash Avenue, Suite 700
Chicago, Illinois 60603
Phone: (312) 346-9813

☐ Northwestern University Cancer
  Center
303 East Chicago Avenue
Chicago, Illinois 60611
Phone: (312) 266-5250

144

☐ University of Chicago Cancer
  Research Center
950 East 59th Street
Chicago, Illinois 60637
Phone: (312) 962-6180

☐ University of Illinois
  Department of Surgery, Division of
    Surgical Oncology
840 South Wood Street
Chicago, Illinois 60612
Phone: (312) 996-6666

☐ Rush Cancer Center
  Suite 820
1725 West Harrison Street
Chicago, Illinois 60612
Phone: (312) 942-6028

MARYLAND
Johns Hopkins Oncology Center
600 North Wolfe Street
Baltimore, Maryland 21205
Phone: (301) 955-8822

MASSACHUSETTS
Dana-Farber Cancer Institute
44 Binney Street
Boston, Massachusetts 02115
Phone: (617) 732-3555

MICHIGAN
Michigan Cancer Foundation
Meyer L. Prentis Cancer Center
110 East Warren Avenue
Detroit, Michigan 48201
Phone: (313) 833-0710

MINNESOTA
Mayo Clinic
200 First Street, S.W.
Rochester, Minnesota 55905
Phone: (507) 284-8964

NEW YORK
Columbia University Cancer
  Research Center
701 West 168th Street, Rm. 1208
New York, New York 10032
Phone: (212) 694-3647

Memorial Sloan-Kettering Cancer
  Center
1275 York Avenue
New York, New York 10021
Phone: (212) 794-6561

Roswell Park Memorial Institute
666 Elm Street
Buffalo, New York 14263
Phone: (716) 845-5770

NORTH CAROLINA
Duke Comprehensive Cancer Center
P.O. Box 3814
Duke University Medical Center
Durham, North Carolina 27710
Phone: (919) 684-2282

OHIO
Ohio State University Comprehen-
  sive Cancer Center
Suite 302
410 West 12th Avenue
Columbus, Ohio, 43210
Phone: (614) 422-5022

PENNSYLVANIA
Fox Chase/University of Pennsylvania
  Cancer Center

☐ The Fox Chase Cancer Center
  7701 Burholme Avenue
Philadelphia, Pennsylvania 19111
Phone: (215) 728-2781

☐ University of Pennsylvania Cancer
  Center
3400 Spruce Street
7th Floor, Silverstein Pavilion
Philadelphia, Pennsylvania 19104
Phone: (215) 662-3910

TEXAS
The University of Texas System Can-
  cer Center
M. D. Anderson Hospital and Tumor
  Institute
6723 Bertner Avenue
Houston, Texas 77030
Phone: (713) 792-6000

WASHINGTON
Fred Hutchinson Cancer Research
 Center
1124 Columbia Street
Seattle, Washington 98104
Phone: (206) 292-2930 or 292-7545

WISCONSIN
Wisconsin Clinical Cancer Center
University of Wisconsin
Department of Human Oncology
600 Highland Avenue
Madison, Wisconsin 53792
Phone: (608) 263-8610

Chartered Divisions of the American Cancer Society, Inc.

Alabama Division, Inc.
402 Office Park Drive
Suite 300
Birmingham, Alabama 35223
Phone: (205) 879-2242

Alaska Division, Inc.
1343 G Street
Anchorage, Alaska 99501
Phone: (907) 277-8696

Arizona Division, Inc.
634 West Indian School Road
P.O. Box 33187
Phoenix, Arizona 85067
Phone: (602) 234-3266

Arkansas Division, Inc.
5520 West Markham Street
P.O. Box 3822
Little Rock, Arkansas 72203
Phone: (501) 664-3480-1-2

California Division, Inc.
1710 Webster Street
P.O. Box 2061
Oakland, California 94604
Phone: (415) 893-7900

Colorado Division, Inc.
2255 South Oneida
P.O. Box 24669
Denver, Colorado 80224
Phone: (303) 758-2030

Connecticut Division, Inc.
Barnes Park South
14 Village Lane
P.O. Box 410
Wallingford, Connecticut 06492
Phone: (203) 265-7161

Delaware Division, Inc.
1708 Lovering Avenue
Suite 202
Wilmington, Delaware 19806
Phone: (302) 654-6267

District of Columbia Division, Inc.
Universal Building, South
1825 Connecticut Avenue, N.W.
Washington, D.C. 20009
Phone: (202) 483-2600

Florida Division, Inc.
1001 South MacDill Avenue
Tampa, Florida 33609
Phone: (813) 253-0541

Georgia Division, Inc.
1422 W. Peachtree Street, N.W.
Atlanta, Georgia 30309
Phone: (404) 892-0026

Hawaii Pacific Division, Inc.
Community Services Center Bldg.
200 North Vineyard Boulevard
Honolulu, Hawaii 96817
Phone: (808) 531-1662-3-4-5

Idaho Division, Inc.
1609 Abbs Street
P.O. Box 5386
Boise, Idaho 83705
Phone: (208) 343-4609

Illinois Division, Inc.
37 South Wabash Avenue
Chicago, Illinois 60603
Phone: (312) 372-0472

Indiana Division, Inc.
9575 N. Valparaiso
Indianapolis, Indiana 46268
Phone: (317) 872-4432

Iowa Division, Inc.
Highway #18 West
P.O. Box 980
Mason City, Iowa 50401
Phone: (515) 423-0712

Kansas Division, Inc.
3003 Van Buren Street
Topeka, Kansas 66611
Phone: (913) 267-0131

Kentucky Division, Inc.
Medical Arts Bldg.
1169 Eastern Parkway
Louisville, Kentucky 40217
Phone: (502) 459-1867

Louisiana Division, Inc.
Masonic Temple Bldg., 7th Floor
333 St. Charles Avenue
New Orleans, Louisiana 70130
Phone: (504) 523-2029

Maine Division, Inc.
Federal and Green Streets
Brunswick, Maine 04011
Phone: (207) 729-3339

Maryland Division, Inc.
1840 York Rd., Suite K–M
P.O. Box 544
Timonium, Maryland 21093
Phone: (301) 561-4790

Massachusetts Division, Inc.
247 Commonwealth Avenue
Boston, Massachusetts 02116
Phone: (617) 267-2650

Michigan Division, Inc.
1205 East Saginaw Street
Lansing, Michigan 48906
Phone: (517) 371-2920

Minnesota Division, Inc.
3316 West 66th Street
Minneapolis, Minnesota 55435
Phone: (612) 925-2772

Mississippi Division, Inc.
345 North Mart Plaza
Jackson, Mississippi 39206
Phone: (601) 362-8874

Missouri Division, Inc.
3322 American Avenue
P.O. Box 1066
Jefferson City, Missouri 65102
Phone: (314) 893-4800

Montana Division, Inc.
2820 First Avenue South
Billings, Montana 59101
Phone: (406) 252-7111

Nebraska Division, Inc.
8502 West Center Road
Omaha, Nebraska 68124
Phone: (402) 393-5800

Nevada Division, Inc.
1325 East Harmon
Las Vegas, Nevada 89109
Phone: (702) 798-6877

New Hampshire Division, Inc.
686 Mast Road
Manchester, New Hampshire 03102
Phone: (603) 669-3270

New Jersey Division, Inc.
CN2201, 2600 Route 1
North Brunswick, New Jersey 08902
Phone: (201) 297-8000

New Mexico Division, Inc.
5800 Lomas Blvd., N.E.
Albuquerque, New Mexico 87110
Phone: (505) 262-2336

New York State Division, Inc.
6725 Lyons Street, P.O. Box 7
East Syracuse, New York 13057
Phone: (315) 437-7025

☐ **Long Island Division, Inc.**
535 Broad Hollow Road
(Route 110)
Melville, New York 11747
Phone: (516) 420-1111

147

☐ New York City Division, Inc.
19 West 56th Street
New York, New York 10019
Phone: (212) 586-8700

☐ Queens Division, Inc.
112-25 Queens Boulevard
Forest Hills, New York 11375
Phone: (212) 263-2224

☐ Westchester Division, Inc.
901 North Broadway
White Plains, New York 10603
Phone: (914) 949-4800

North Carolina Division, Inc.
11 South Boylan Avenue
Suite 221
Raleigh, North Carolina 27603
Phone: (919) 834-8463

North Dakota Division, Inc.
Hotel Graver Annex Bldg.
115 Roberts Street
P.O. Box 426
Fargo, North Dakota 58102
Phone: (701) 232-1385

Ohio Division, Inc.
1375 Euclid Avenue
Suite 312
Cleveland, Ohio 44115
Phone: (216) 771-6700

Oklahoma Division, Inc.
3800 North Cromwell
Oklahoma City, Oklahoma 73112
Phone: (405) 946-5000

Oregon Division, Inc.
0330 S.W. Curry
Portland, Oregon 97201
Phone: (503) 295-6422

Pennsylvania Division, Inc.
Route 422 & Sipe Avenue
P.O. Box 416
Hershey, Pennsylvania 17033
Phone: (717) 533-6144

☐ Philadelphia Division, Inc.
1422 Chestnut Street
Philadelphia, Pennsylvania 19102
Phone: (215) 665-2900

Puerto Rico Division, Inc.
(Avenue Domenech 273
Hato Rey, P.R.)
GPO Box 6004
San Juan, Puerto Rico 00936
Phone: (809) 764-2295

Rhode Island Division, Inc.
345 Blackstone Blvd.
Providence, Rhode Island 02906
Phone: (401) 831-6970

South Carolina Division, Inc.
2442 Devine Street
Columbia, South Carolina 29205
Phone: (803) 256-0245

South Dakota Division, Inc.
1025 North Minnesota Avenue
Hillcrest Plaza
Sioux Falls, South Dakota 57104
Phone: (605) 336-0897

Tennessee Division, Inc.
713 Melpark Drive
Nashville, Tennessee 37204
Phone: (615) 383-1710

Texas Division, Inc.
3834 Spicewood Springs Road
P.O. Box 9863
Austin, Texas 78766
Phone: (512) 345-4560

Utah Division, Inc.
610 East South Temple
Salt Lake City, Utah 84102
Phone: (801) 322-0431

Vermont Division, Inc.
13 Loomis Street, Drawer C
Montpelier, Vermont 05602
Phone: (802) 223-2348

Virginia Division, Inc.
4240 Park Place Court
P.O. Box 1547
Glen Allen, Virginia 23060
Phone: (804) 270-0142

Washington Division, Inc.
2120 First Avenue North
Seattle, Washington 98109
Phone: (206) 283-1152

West Virginia Division, Inc.
Suite 100
240 Capitol Street
Charleston, West Virginia 25301
Phone: (304) 344-3611

Wisconsin Division, Inc.
615 North Sherman Avenue
P.O. Box 8370
Madison, Wisconsin 53708
Phone: (608) 249-0487

☐ Milwaukee Division, Inc.
11401 West Watertown Plank Road
Wauwatosa, Wisconsin 53226
Phone: (414) 453-4500

Wyoming Division, Inc.
Indian Hills Center
506 Shoshoni
Cheyenne, Wyoming 82009
Phone: (307) 638-3331

NATIONAL HEADQUARTERS:
AMERICAN CANCER SOCIETY, INC.,
90 PARK AVENUE
NEW YORK, N.Y., 10016

Association of American Cancer Institutes
Clinical Cancer Centers

The following institutions have met the requirements for admission to, and are members of the Association of American Cancer Institutes:

ARIZONA
University of Arizona Cancer Center
University of Arizona
College of Medicine
Tucson, Arizona 85724
Phone: (602) 626-6044

CALIFORNIA
Northern California Cancer Program
1801 Page Mill Road
Building B, Suite 200
P.O. Box 10144
Palo Alto, California 94303
Phone: (415) 497-5877

California Research Institute
University of California
San Francisco, California 94143

University of California
San Diego Cancer Center
School of Medicine
La Jolla, California 92093
Phone: (619) 294-6930

Cancer Research Center
City of Hope Research Institute
1450 East Duarte Road
Duarte, California 91010
Phone: (213) 357-9711, Ext. 2705

COLORADO
AMC Cancer Research Center &
    Hospital
6401 W. Colfax Avenue
Lakewood, Colorado 80214

149

GEORGIA
Emory University Cancer Center
Emory University Hospital
Atlanta, Georgia 30322

HAWAII
Cancer Center of Hawaii
University of Hawaii at Manoa
1236 Lauhala Street
Honolulu, Hawaii 96813
Phone: (808) 548-8415 or 8416

IDAHO
Mountain States Tumor Institute
151 East Bannock
Boise, Idaho 83702

IOWA
University of Iowa Cancer Center
College of Medicine
20 Medical Laboratories
Iowa City, Iowa 55242
Phone: (319) 353-6595

KENTUCKY
James Graham Brown Cancer Center
529 South Jackson Street
Louisville, Kentucky 40202

MASSACHUSETTS
Tufts-New England Medical Center
Box 842
171 Harrison Avenue
Boston, Massachusetts 02111
Phone: (617) 956-5406

New England Deaconess Cancer
   Research Institute
185 Pilgrim Road
Boston, Massachusetts 02215

MISSOURI
Ellis Fischel Cancer Center
Business Loop 70 & Garth Avenue
Columbia, Missouri 65205

NEBRASKA
Eppley Institute for Research in
   Cancer
42nd & Dewey Avenue
Omaha, Nebraska 68105

NEW HAMPSHIRE
Norris Cotton Cancer Center
Dartmouth-Hitchcock Medical Center
Hanover, New Hampshire 03755
Phone: (603) 646-5505

NEW JERSEY
Institute for Medical Research
Copewood Street
Camden, New Jersey 08103

NEW MEXICO
Cancer Research & Treatment Center
University of New Mexico
900 Camino De Salud NE
Albuquerque, New Mexico 87131

NEW YORK
Mt. Sinai Cancer Center
Fifth Avenue at 100th Street
New York, New York 10029
Phone: (212) 650-6361

Albert Einstein Cancer Research
   Center
1300 Morris Park Avenue
Bronx, New York 10461
Phone: (212) 430-2302

New York University Cancer Center
55 First Avenue
New York, New York 10016
Phone: (212) 340-5349

University of Rochester Cancer
   Center
601 Elmwood Avenue, Box 704
Rochester, New York 14642
Phone: (716) 275-4865

NORTH CAROLINA
Cancer Research Center
University of North Carolina
Box 30
MacNider Building 202H
Chapel Hill, North Carolina 27514
Phone: (919) 966-1183 or 3036

Oncology Research Center
Bowman Gray School of Medicine
300 South Hawthorne Road
Winston-Salem, North Carolina 27103
Phone: (919) 748-4606

OHIO
Cleveland Clinic Cancer Center
9500 Euclid Avenue
Cleveland, Ohio 44106

PENNSYLVANIA
Hahnemann Cancer Institute
230 North Brook Street
Philadelphia, Pennsylvania 19102

Clinical Radiation Therapy Research
Center
Allegheny General Hospital
328 East North Avenue
Pittsburgh, Pennsylvania 15212

Childrens Cancer Research Center
34th and Arie Center Civic Blvd.
Philadelphia, Pennsylvania 19104

PUERTO RICO
I. Gonzalez Martinez Oncologic
Hospital
Puerto Rico Medical Center
Hato Rey, Puerto Rico 00919

Puerto Rico Cancer Center
University of Puerto Rico
Medical Sciences Campus
G.P.O. Box 5067
San Juan, Puerto Rico 00936
Phone: (809) 751-6242

Hospital Oncologico
Centro Medico de Ponce
Ponce, Puerto Rico 00733

RHODE ISLAND
Brown University Cancer Center
Roger Williams General Hospital
825 Chalkstone Avenue
Providence, Rhode Island 02908
Phone: (401) 456-2070

TENNESSEE
Memphis Regional Cancer Center
3 North Dunlop
Memphis, Tennessee 38163

St. Jude Children's Research Hospital
332 North Lauderdale
Memphis, Tennessee 38101
Phone: (901) 522-0301

TEXAS
UTMB Cancer Center
University of Texas Medical Branch
Galveston, Texas 77550
Phone: (713) 765-2981

VERMONT
Vermont Regional Cancer Center
University of Vermont
1 South Prospect Street
Burlington, Vermont 95401
Phone: (802) 656-4414

VIRGINIA
MCV/VCU Cancer Center
MCV Box 37
Medical College of Virginia
Virginia Commonwealth University
Richmond, Virginia 23298
Phone: (804) 786-9322/9323 or
   786-0448

~Appendix 2~

<u>Cancer Programs Approved by the Commission on Cancer of the American College of Surgeons</u>

ALABAMA
Birmingham
   AMI Brockwood Medical Center
   Baptist Medical Center—Montclair
   Baptist Medical Center—Princeton
   Carraway Methodist Medical
     Center
   St. Vincent's Hospital
   University of Alabama Hospitals
   Veterans Administration Medical
     Center
Gadsden
   Baptist Memorial Hospital
Mobile
   Mobile Infirmary Medical Center
   University of South Alabama
     Medical Center
Selma
   Selma Medical Center
Tuskegee
   Veterans Administration Medical
     Center

ALASKA
Fairbanks
   Fairbanks Memorial Hospital

ARIZONA
Mesa
   Desert Samaritan Hospital
   Mesa Lutheran Hospital
Phoenix
   Good Samaritan Medical
     Center
   Maricopa Medical Center
   Phoenix Memorial Hospital
   Veterans Administration Medical
     Center
Scottsdale
   Scottsdale Memorial Hospital
Tucson
   Tucson Medical Center
   University Medical Center

153

Appendix 2

ARKANSAS

Fayetteville
  Washington Regional Medical
    Center
Fort Smith
  Sparks Regional Medical Center
  St. Edward Mercy Medical Center
Little Rock
  John L. McClellan Memorial
    Veterans Hospital
  St. Vincent Infirmary
  University Hospital of Arkansas
Rogers
  St. Mary–Rogers Memorial
    Hospital

CALIFORNIA

Alhambra
  Alhambra Community Hospital
Anaheim
  Anaheim Memorial Hospital
  Humana Hospital—West Anaheim
  Martin Luther Hospital Medical
    Center
Apple Valley
  St. Mary Desert Valley Hospital
Arcadia
  Methodist Hospital of Southern
    California
Bakersfield
  Kern Medical Center
  San Joaquin Community Hospital
Bellflower
  Bellwood General Hospital
  Kaiser Foundation Hospital (RCS)
Berkeley
  Alta Bates Hospital
  Herrick Hospital & Health Center
Burbank
  St. Joseph Medical Center
Burlingame
  Peninsula Hospital & Medical
    Center
Castro Valley
  Eden Hospital Medical Center
Chico
  N. T. Enloe Memorial Hospital
Concord
  Mount Diablo Hospital Medical
    Center

Covina
  Inter-Community Medical Center
Daly City
  Seton Medical Center
Downey
  Downey Community Hospital
Duarte
  City of Hope National Medical
    Center
  Santa Teresita Hospital
Encino
  Encino Hospital
Escondido
  Palomar Memorial Hospital
Fontana
  Kaiser Foundation Hospital (SIE)
Fountain Valley
  Fountain Valley Regional Medical
    Center
Fresno
  Fresno Community Hospital &
    Medical Center
  St. Agnes Hospital & Medical
    Center
  Valley Children's Hospital
  Veterans Administration Medical
    Center
Fullerton
  St. Jude Hospital—Fullerton
Glendale
  Glendale Adventist Medical Center
  Glendale Memorial Hospital &
    Health Center
Glendora
  AMI Glendora Community
    Hospital
  Foothill Presbyterian Hospital
Granada Hills
  Granada Hills Community Hospital
Harbor City
  Bay Harbor Hospital
  Kaiser Foundation Hospital (VER)
Hawthorne
  Robert F. Kennedy Medical Center
Indio
  John F. Kennedy Memorial Hospital
Inglewood
  Centinela Hospital Medical Center
  Daniel Freeman Memorial Hospital
La Jolla
  Green Hospital of Scripps College

Scripps Memorial Hospital—La
Jolla
La Mesa
Grossmont District Hospital
La Palma
La Palma Intercommunity
Hospital
Laguna Hills
Saddleback Hospital & Health
Center
Lakewood
Doctors Hospital of Lakewood—
South St.
Loma Linda
Loma Linda University Medical
Center
Long Beach
Long Beach Community Hospital
Memorial Medical Center
St. Mary Medical Center
Veterans Administration Medical
Center
Los Alamitos
Los Alamitos Medical Center
Los Angeles
California Medical Center—Los
Angeles
Cedars-Sinai Medical Center
Childrens Hospital of Los Angeles
Cigna Hospital of Los Angeles
Hollywood Presbyterian Medical
Center
Hospital of the Good Samaritan
Kaiser Foundation Hospital (CAD)
Kaiser Foundation Hospital (SUN)
Los Angeles County—USC Medical
Center
Martin Luther King Jr. General
Hospital
Orthopaedic Hospital
Queen of Angels Medical Center
Santa Marta Hospital
St. Vincent Medical Center
University of California at Los
Angeles Medical Center
USC—Kenneth Norris Jr. Cancer
Hospital
White Memorial Medical Center
Martinez
Veterans Administration Medical
Center

Mission Viejo
Mission Hospital Regional Medical
Center
Modesto
Memorial Hospitals Association
Montebello
Beverly Hospital
Monterey Park
Garfield Medical Center
Monterey Park Hospital
Napa
Napa State Hospital
Queen of the Valley Hospital
National City
Paradise Valley Hospital
Newport Beach
Hoag Memorial Hospital
Presbyterian
Northridge
Northridge Hospital Medical
Center
Oakland
Naval Hospital
Samuel Merritt Hospital
Oceanside
Tri-City Medical Center
Orange
Childrens Hospital of Orange
St. Joseph Hospital
University of California Irvine
Medical Center
Oxnard
St. John's Hospital Regional Medical
Center
Palm Springs
Desert Hospital
Palo Alto
Veterans Administration Medical
Center
Panorama City
Kaiser Foundation Hospital (CAN)
Pasadena
Huntington Memorial Hospital
St. Luke Medical Center
Pomona
Pomona Valley Community
Hospital
Poway
Pomerado Hospital
Rancho Mirage
Eisenhower Medical Center

CALIFORNIA (*Cont.*)

Redding
Mercy Medical Center

Redlands
Redlands Community Hospital

Redondo Beach
AMI South Bay Hospital

Redwood City
Sequoia Hospital District

Riverside
Parkview Community Hospital
Riverside Community Hospital

Sacramento
Mercy Hospital of Sacramento
Sutter Community Hospitals
University of California Davis
Medical Center

San Bernardino
San Bernardino Community
Hospital
San Bernardino County Medical
Center
St. Bernardine Medical Center

San Clemente
San Clemente General Hospital

San Diego
Children's Hospital & Health
Center
Kaiser Foundation Hospital (ZIO)
Naval Hospital
Sharp Memorial Hospital
University of California San Diego
Medical Center

San Dimas
AMI San Dimas Community
Hospital

San Francisco
Children's Hospital of San
Francisco
French Hospital
Letterman Army Medical Center
Marshal Hale Memorial Hospital
Mount Zion Hospital & Medical
Center
Pacific Presbyterian Medical
Center
Ralph K. Davies Medical Center
St. Francis Memorial Hospital
St. Luke's Hospital
St. Mary's Hospital & Medical
Center

University of California San
Francisco Medical Center

San Gabriel
San Gabriel Valley Medical Center

San Jose
Good Samaritan Hospital
O'Connor Hospital
San Jose Hospital
Santa Clara Valley Medical Center

San Pablo
Brookside Hospital

San Pedro
San Pedro Peninsula Hospital

San Rafael
Marin General Hospital

Santa Ana
Western Medical Center

Santa Barbara
Goleta Valley Community
Hospital
Santa Barbara Cottage Hospital
St. Francis Hospital of Santa
Barbara

Santa Cruz
Dominican Santa Cruz Hospital

Santa Monica
Santa Monica Hospital Medical
Center
St. John's Hospital & Health Center

South Laguna
South Coast Medical Center

Stockton
Dameron Hospital
St. Joseph's Medical Center

Tarzana
AMI Tarzana Regional Medical
Center

Thousand Oaks
Los Robles Regional Medical
Center

Torrance
LAC-Harbor—University of
California at LAMC
Little Company of Mary Hospital
Torrance Memorial Hospital
Medical Center

Travis Air Force Base
David Grant U.S. Air Force Medical
Center

Upland
San Antonio Community Hospital

Van Nuys
 Valley Presbyterian Hospital
Victorville
 Victor Valley Community Hospital
Visalia
 Kaweah Delta District Hospital
Walnut Creek
 John Muir Memorial Hospital
West Covina
 Queen of the Valley Hospital
Whittier
 Presbyterian Intercommunity
  Hospital

COLORADO
Aurora
 Fitzsimons Army Medical Center
Colorado Springs
 Penrose Hospitals
Denver
 AMI Presbyterian Denver Hospital
 AMI St. Luke's Hospital
 Porter Memorial Hospital
 Rose Medical Center
 St. Joseph Hospital
 University Hospital
 Veterans Administration Medical
  Center
Englewood
 Swedish Medical Center
Fort Carson
 U.S. Army Community Hospital
Fort Collins
 Poudre Valley Hospital
Greeley
 North Colorado Medical Center
Lakewood
 AMC Cancer Research Center
Longmont
 Longmont United Hospital
Montrose
 Montrose Memorial Hospital
Pueblo
 St. Mary-Corwin Hospital
Wheat Ridge
 Lutheran Medical Center

CONNECTICUT
Bridgeport
 Bridgeport Hospital

 Park City Hospital
 St. Vincent's Medical Center
Bristol
 Bristol Hospital
Danbury
 Danbury Hospital
Derby
 Griffin Hospital
Farmington
 John Dempsey Hospital University
  of Connecticut
Greenwich
 Greenwich Hospital
Hartford
 Hartford Hospital
 Mount Sinai Hospital
 St. Francis Hospital & Medical
  Center
Meriden
 Meriden–Wallingford Hospital
Middletown
 Middlesex Memorial Hospital
New Haven
 Hospital of St. Raphael
 Yale–New Haven Hospital
Norwalk
 Norwalk Hospital
Sharon
 Sharon Hospital
Stamford
 St. Joseph Medical Center
 Stamford Hospital
Torrington
 Charlotte Hungerford Hospital
Waterbury
 St. Mary's Hospital
 Waterbury Hospital

DELAWARE
Dover
 Kent General Hospital
Lewes
 Beebe Hospital of Sussex County
Wilmington
 Medical Center of Delaware
 St. Francis Hospital

DISTRICT OF COLUMBIA
Washington, D.C.
 Georgetown University Medical
  Center

DIST. OF COLUMBIA (*Cont*)

Washington, D.C.
  Greater Southeast Community
    Hospital
  Howard University Hospital
  Veterans Administration Medical
    Center
  Walter Reed Army Medical
    Center
  Washington Hospital Center

FLORIDA

Boca Raton
  Boca Raton Community Hospital
Bradenton
  Manatee Memorial Hospital
Clearwater
  Morton F. Plant Hospital
Daytona Beach
  Halifax Hospital Medical Center
Dunedin
  Mease Hospital Dunedin
Fort Lauderdale
  Broward General Medical
    Center
Fort Myers
  Lee Memorial Hospital
  Southwest Florida Regional
    Medical Center
Gainesville
  Shands Hospital at the University
    of Florida
Jacksonville
  Jacksonville Wolfson Childrens
    Hospital
  Naval Hospital
  St. Vincent's Medical Center
  University Hospital of Jacksonville
Largo
  HCA Largo Medical Center
    Hospital
Miami
  Baptist Hospital of Miami
  Cedars Medical Center
  James M. Jackson Memorial
    Hospital
  North Shore Medical Center
Miami Beach
  Mount Sinai Medical Center
Naples
  Naples Community Hospital

Ocala
  Marion Community Hospital
  Munroe Regional Medical Center
Orlando
  Orlando Regional Medical Center
Pensacola
  Baptist Hospital
  Naval Hospital
  Sacred Heart Hospital of
    Pensacola
  West Florida Medical Center
South Miami
  South Miami Hospital
St. Petersburg
  Bayfront Medical Center
Stuart
  Martin Memorial Hospital
Tallahassee
  Tallahassee Memorial Regional
    Medical Center
Tampa
  St. Joseph's Hospital
  Tampa General Hospital
  University Community Hospital

GEORGIA

Americus
  Sumter Regional Hospital
Atlanta
  Crawford Long Hospital of Emory
    University
  Emory University Hospital
  Georgia Baptist Medical Center
  HCA West Paces Ferry Hospital
  Northside Hospital
  Piedmont Hospital
  St. Joseph's Hospital
Augusta
  Medical College of Georgia
    Hospital
  University Hospital
Austell
  Cobb General Hospital
Columbus
  Medical Center
Conyers
  Rockdale Hospital
Dalton
  Hamilton Medical Center
Decatur
  Dekalb General Hospital

Veterans Administration Medical
  Center Atlanta
Dublin
  Fairview Park Hospital
East Point
  South Fulton Hospital
Fort Benning
  Martin Army Community Hospital
Fort Gordon
  Dwight D. Eisenhower Army
    Medical Center
Gainesville
  Northeast Georgia Medical Center
Jesup
  Wayne Memorial Hospital
La Grange
  West Georgia Medical Center
Marietta
  Kennestone Hospital
Rome
  Floyd Medical Center
Savannah
  Memorial Medical Center
Snellville
  Humana Hospital—Gwinnett
Statesboro
  Bulloch Memorial Hospital
Valdosta
  South Georgia Medical Center

HAWAII
Honolulu
  Kaiser Foundation Hospital
  Kuakini Medical Center
  Queen's Medical Center
  St. Francis Medical Center
  Straub Clinic and Hospital
  Tripler Army Medical Center
Lihue
  G. N. Wilcox Memorial Hospital
Wailuku
  Maui Memorial Hospital
Waimea
  Kauai Veterans Memorial Hospital

IDAHO
Blackfoot
  Bingham Memorial Hospital
Boise
  St. Alphonsus Regional Medical
    Center

St. Luke's Regional Medical Center
Burley
  Cassia Memorial Hospital &
    Medical Center
Lewiston
  St. Joseph Regional Medical Center
Nampa
  Mercy Medical Center
Pocatello
  Bannock Regional Medical Center
  Pocatello Regional Medical Center
Twin Falls
  Magic Valley Regional Medical
    Center

ILLINOIS
Arlington Heights
  Northwest Community Hospital
Aurora
  Copley Memorial Hospital
  Mercy Center for Health Care
    Service
Barrington
  Good Shepherd Hospital
Belleville
  Memorial Hospital
  St. Elizabeth's Hospital
Berwyn
  MacNeal Hospital
Blue Island
  St. Francis Hospital
Carbondale
  Memorial Hospital
Centralia
  St. Mary's Hospital
Champaign
  Burnham Hospital
Chicago
  Central Community Hospital
  Children's Memorial Hospital
  Columbus Hospital
  Cook County Hospital
  Edgewater Hospital
  Franklin Boulevard Community
    Hospital
  Grant Hospital of Chicago
  Holy Cross Hospital
  Illinois Masonic Medical Center
  Jackson Park Hospital
  John F. Kennedy Medical Center
  Louis A. Weiss Memorial Hospital

159

ILLINOIS (*Cont.*)

Chicago
Lutheran General Hospital—
Lincoln Park
Mary Thompson Hospital
Mercy Hospital & Medical Center
Methodist Hospital of Chicago
Michael Reese Hospital & Medical
Center
Mount Sinai Hospital Medical
Center
Northwestern Memorial Hospital
Ravenswood Hospital Medical
Center
Resurrection Hospital
Rush–Presbyterian–St. Luke's
Medical Center
South Chicago Community
Hospital
St. Elizabeth's Hospital
St. Mary of Nazareth Hospital
Center
Swedish Covenant Hospital
University of Chicago Hospitals
University of Illinois Hospital
Veterans Administration West Side
Medical Center
Chicago Heights
St. James Hospital Medical Center
Danville
Lakeview Medical Center
St. Elizabeth Hospital
De Kalb
Kishwaukee Community Hospital
Decatur
Decatur Memorial Hospital
St. Mary's Hospital
Des Plaines
Holy Family Hospital
Dixon
Katherine Shaw Bethea Hospital
Downers Grove
Good Samaritan Hospital
Effingham
St. Anthony's Memorial Hospital
Elgin
Sherman Hospital
St. Joseph Hospital
Elk Grove Village
Alexian Brothers Medical
Center

Elmhurst
Elmhurst Memorial Hospital
Evanston
Evanston Hospital
St. Francis Hospital
Evergreen Park
Little Company of Mary Hospital
Galesburg
St. Mary's Hospital
Granite City
St. Elizabeth Medical Center
Great Lakes
Naval Hospital
Harvey
Ingalls Memorial Hospital
Hazel Crest
South Suburban Hospital
Highland Park
Highland Park Hospital
Hinsdale
Hinsdale Hospital
Joliet
Silver Cross Hospital
St. Joseph Medical Center
Kankakee
St. Mary's Hospital of Kankakee
La Grange
La Grange Memorial Hospital
Lake Forest
Lake Forest Hospital
Libertyville
Condell Memorial Hospital
Macomb
McDonough District Hospital
Maywood
Foster G. McGaw Hospital
McHenry
Northern Illinois Medical Center
Moline
Lutheran Hospital
Morris
Morris Hospital
Mount Vernon
Good Samaritan Hospital
Naperville
Edward Hospital
Oak Lawn
Christ Hospital & Medical Center
Oak Park
West Suburban Hospital Medical
Center

Olney
　Richland Memorial Hospital
Park Ridge
　Lutheran General Hospital
Peoria
　Methodist Medical Center of
　　Illinois
　St. Francis Medical Center
Pontiac
　St. James Hospital
Quincy
　Blessing Hospital
　St. Mary Hospital
Rockford
　Rockford Memorial Hospital
　St. Anthony Medical Center
　Swedish-American Hospital
Skokie
　Rush North Shore Medical Center
Springfield
　Memorial Medical Center
　St. John's Hospital
Sterling
　Community General Hospital
Ureana
　Carle Foundation Hospital
　Mercy Hospital
Waukegan
　St. Therese Medical Center
　Victory Memorial Hospital
Winfield
　Central DuPage Hospital
Zion
　American International Hospital

INDIANA
Bluffton
　Caylor-Nickel Hospital
Columbus
　Bartholomew County Hospital
Evansville
　Deaconess Hospital
　St. Mary's Medical Center
　Welborn Memorial Baptist Hospital
Gary
　Methodist Hospital of Northwest
　　Indiana
Hammond
　St. Margaret Hospital
Indianapolis
　Community Hospitals of Indiana

　Methodist Hospital of Indiana
　St. Vincent Hospital
Lafayette
　St. Elizabeth Hospital Medical
　　Center
New Albany
　Floyd Memorial Hospital
South Bend
　Memorial Hospital of South Bend
　St. Joseph's Medical Center
Terre Haute
　Terre Haute Regional Hospital
　Union Hospital
Vincennes
　Good Samaritan Hospital

IOWA
Des Moines
　Iowa Methodist Medical Center
　Mercy Hospital Medical Center
　Veterans Administration Medical
　　Center
Iowa City
　University of Iowa Hospitals
Mason City
　North Iowa Medical Center
　St. Joseph Mercy Hospital
Sioux City
　Marian Health Center
　St. Luke's Regional Medical Center

KANSAS
Fort Riley
　Irwin Army Community Hospital
Hays
　Hadley Regional Medical Center
　St. Anthony Hospital
Kansas City
　Bethany Medical Center
　Providence–St. Margaret Health
　University of Kansas Hospital
Shawnee Mission
　Shawnee Mission Medical Center
Topeka
　St. Francis Hospital & Medical
　　Center
Wichita
　HCA Wesley Medical Center
　St. Francis Regional Medical
　　Center
　St. Joseph Medical Center

KENTUCKY

Fort Campbell
Col. F. A. Blanchfield Army
    Community Hospital
Fort Thomas
St. Luke Hospital
Lexington
Central Baptist Hospital
Good Samaritan Hospital
University Hospital
Louisville
Baptist Hospital East
Baptist Hospital Highlands
Humana Hospital–University
Kosair/Children's Hospital
Norton Hospital
Veterans Administration Medical
    Center
Madisonville
Regional Medical Center

LOUISIANA

Alexandria
Rapides General Hospital
St. Frances Cabrini Hospital
Lafayette
University Medical Center
Lake Charles
St. Patrick Hospital
New Orleans
Charity Hospital of New Orleans
Ochsner Foundation Hospital
Touro Infirmary
Veterans Administration Medical
    Center
Shreveport
Louisiana State University Hospital
Veterans Administration Medical
    Center

MAINE

Augusta
Kennebec Valley Medical Center
Bangor
Eastern Maine Medical Center
Lewiston
Central Maine Medical Center
St. Mary's General Hospital
Portland
Maine Medical Center

Rockland
Penobscot Bay Medical Center
Rumford
Rumford Community Hospital
Skowhegan
Redington-Fairview General
    Hospital
Togus
Veterans Administration Medical
    Center
Waterville
Mid-Maine Medical Center

MARYLAND

Annapolis
Anne Arundel General Hospital
Baltimore
Johns Hopkins Hospital
Sinai Hospital of Baltimore
St. Agnes Hospital
University of Maryland Medical
    Systems
Bethesda
Naval Hospital
Cumberland
Sacred Heart Hospital
Frederick
Frederick Memorial Hospital
Hagerstown
Washington County Hospital
Olney
Montgomery General Hospital
Salisbury
Peninsula General Hospital
    Medical Center
Takona Park
Washington Adventist Hospital

MASSACHUSETTS

Arlington
Choate-Symmes Health Services
Beverly
Beverly Hospital
Boston
Boston City Hospital
Brigham & Women's Hospital
Carney Hospital
Children's Hospital
Faulkner Hospital
Massachusetts General Hospital

New England Deaconess Hospital
New England Medical Center
University Hospital
Brighton
St. Elizabeth's Hospital of Boston
Brockton
Brockton Hospital
Cardinal Cushing General Hospital
Burlington
Lahey Clinic Hospital
Cambridge
Mount Auburn Hospital
Chelsea
Lawrence F. Quigley Memorial
Hospital
Concord
Emerson Hospital
Danvers
Hunt Memorial Hospital
Fall River
Charlton Memorial Hospital
St. Anne's Hospital
Framingham
Framingham Union Hospital
Gloucester
Addison Gilbert Hospital
Greenfield
Franklin Medical Center
Holyoke
Holyoke Hospital
Providence Hospital
Hyannis
Cape Cod Hospital
Jamaica Plain, Boston
Veterans Administration Medical
Center
Lowell
Lowell General Hospital
St. John's Hospital
St. Joseph's Hospital
Lynn
Atlanticare Medical Center
Malden
Malden Hospital
Melrose
Melrose–Wakefield Hospital
Association
Natick
Leonard Morse Hospital
Needham
Glover Memorial Hospital

Newton
Newton–Wellesley Hospital
Norfolk
Southwood Community Hospital
North Adams
North Adams Regional Hospital
Northampton
Cooley Dickinson Hospital
Norwood
Norwood Hospital
Palmer
Wing Memorial Hospital & Medical
Centers
Pittsfield
Berkshire Medical Center
Plymouth
Jordan Hospital
Salem
Salem Hospital
South Weymouth
South Shore Hospital
Springfield
Baystate Medical Center
Mercy Hospital
Stoneham
New England Memorial Hospital
Stoughton
Goddard Memorial Hospital
Turners Falls
Farren Memorial Hospital
Waltham
Waltham Weston Hospital &
Medical Center
Winchester
Winchester Hospital
Worcester
St. Vincent Hospital
University of Massachusetts
Medical Center
Worcester Memorial Hospital

MICHIGAN
Allen Park
Veterans Administration Medical
Center
Ann Arbor
University of Michigan Medical
Center
Battle Creek
Leila Hospital & Health
Center

163

MICHIGAN (*Cont.*)
Bay City
Bay Medical Center
Dearborn
Oakwood Hospital
Detroit
Harper-Grace Hospital
Henry Ford Hospital
Flint
Hurley Medical Center
St. Joseph Hospital
Grand Rapids
Blodgett Memorial Medical
Center
Butterworth Hospital
Ferguson Hospital
St. Mary's Health Services
Kalamazoo
Borgess Medical Center
Bronson Methodist Hospital
Lansing
Edward W. Sparrow Hospital
St. Lawrence Hospital
Marquette
Marquette General Hospital
Midland
Midland Hospital Center
Muskegon
Hackley Hospital
Petoskey
Northern Michigan Hospitals
Rochester
Crittenton Hospital
Royal Oak
William Beaumont Hospital
Saginaw
St. Mary's Hospital
Southfield
Providence Hospital
Traverse City
Munson Medical Center
Warren
Macomb Hospital Center

MINNESOTA
Fridley
Unity Medical Center
Grand Rapids
Itasca Memorial Hospital
Mankato
Immanuel–St. Joseph's Hospital

Minneapolis
Abbott-Northwestern Hospital
Hennepin County Medical Center
Methodist Hospital
Metropolitan Medical Center
Minneapolis Childrens Medical
Center
St. Mary's Hospital Division
Veterans Administration Medical
Center
Moorhead
St. Ansgar Hospital
Robbinsdale
North Memorial Medical Center
Rochester
Mayo Clinic
St. Paul
St. Joseph's Hospital Division
St. Paul–Ramsey Medical Center

MISSISSIPPI
Biloxi
Biloxi Regional Medical Center
Veterans Administration Medical
Center
Hattiesburg
Forrest County General Hospital
Methodist Hospital of Hattiesburg
Jackson
Mississippi Baptist Medical Center
University Hospital
Veterans Administration Medical
Center
Keesler Air Force Base
U.S. Air Force Medical Center
Keesler
Oxford
Oxford–Lafayette Medical Center
Pascagoula
Singing River Hospital System
Tupelo
North Mississippi Medical Center
Vicksburg
Mercy Regional Medical Center

MISSOURI
Cape Girardeal
Southeast Missouri Hospital
St. Francis Medical Center
Chesterfield
St. Luke's Hospital

Columbia
AMI Columbia Regional Hospital
Boone Hospital Center
Ellis Fischel State Cancer Center
University of Missouri–Columbia
Hospital & Clinics
Fort Leonard Wood
Gen. Leonard Wood Army
Community Hospital
Jefferson City
Memorial Community Hospital
Joplin
St. John's Regional Medical Center
Kansas City
Baptist Medical Center
Children's Mercy Hospital
Menorah Medical Center
Research Medical Center
St. Joseph Health Center of Kansas
City
St. Luke's Hospital
Trinity Lutheran Hospital
Truman Medical Center—West
Poplar Bluff
Doctors Regional Medical Center
Sikeston
Missouri Delta Medical Center
Springfield
Lester E. Cox Medical Centers
St. Joseph
Heartland Hospital West
St. Louis
Barnes Hospital
Christian Hospitals NE/NW
Deaconess Hospital
Jewish Hospital of St. Louis
St. Anthony's Medical Center
St. John's Mercy Medical Center
St. Mary's Health Center
Veterans Administration Medical
Center—JC Division

MONTANA
Great Falls
Columbus Hospital

NEBRASKA
Hastings
Mary Lanning Memorial Hospital
Kearney
Good Samaritan Hospital

Lincoln
Bryan Memorial Hospital
Lincoln General Hospital
St. Elizabeth Community Health
Center
Veterans Administration Medical
Center
Omaha
AMI St. Joseph Hospital
Archbishop Bergan Mercy Hospital
Bishop Clarkson Memorial
Hospital
Immanuel Medical Center
Lutheran Medical Center
Methodist Hospital
University Hospital–University of
Nebraska
Scottsbluff
West Nebraska General Hospital

NEVADA
Las Vegas
Humana Hospital—Sunrise
University Medical Center of
Southern Nevada
Reno
Washoe Medical Center

NEW HAMPSHIRE
Concord
Concord Hospital
Dover
Wentworth-Douglass Hospital
Exeter
Exeter Hospital
Hanover
Mary Hitchcock Memorial Hospital
Keene
Cheshire Medical Center
Laconia
Lakes Region General Hospital
Littleton
Littleton Hospital
Manchester
Catholic Medical Center
Elliot Hospital
Veterans Administration Medical
Center
Portsmouth
Portsmouth Regional Hospital

165

NEW HAMPSHIRE (*Cont.*)
Rochester
Frisbie Memorial Hospital
Woodsville
Cottage Hospital

NEW JERSEY
Atlantic City
Atlantic City Medical Center
Belleville
Clara Maass Medical Center
Camden
West Jersey Hospital, Northern
Division
Denville
St. Clare's–Riverside Medical
Center
Dover
Dover General Hospital & Medical
Center
East Orange
Veterans Administration Medical
Center
Edison
John F. Kennedy Medical Center
Elizabeth
Elizabeth General Medical Center
St. Elizabeth Hospital
Englewood
Englewood Hospital
Hackensack
Hackensack Medical Center
Hackettstown
Hackettstown Community Hospital
Livingston
St. Barnabas Medical Center
Long Branch
Monmouth Medical Center
Montclair
Mountainside Hospital
Morristown
Morristown Memorial Hospital
Mount Holly
Memorial Hospital of Burlington
County
Neptune
Jersey Shore Medical Center
New Brunswick
Robert Wood Johnson University
Hospital

St. Peter's Medical Center
Newark
Newark Beth Israel Medical Center
University Hospital
Newton
Newton Memorial Hospital
Orange
Hospital Center at Orange
Passaic
Beth Israel Hospital
General Hospital Center at Passaic
Paterson
St. Joseph's Hospital & Medical
Center
Phillipsburg
Warren Hospital
Princeton
Medical Center at Princeton
Red Bank
Riverview Medical Center
Ridgewood
Valley Hospital
Somerville
Somerset Medical Center
Summit
Overlook Hospital
Sussex
Wallkill Valley General Hospital
Teaneck
Holy Name Hospital
Toms River
Community Memorial Hospital
Trenton
Mercer Medical Center
St. Francis Medical Center
Vineland
Newcomb Medical Center
Westwood
Pascack Valley Hospital

NEW MEXICO
Albuquerque
Lovelace Medical Center
Presbyterian Hospital
St. Joseph Health Care Corporation
University of New Mexico Hospital
Veterans Administration Medical
Center
Santa Fe
St. Vincent Hospital

NEW YORK

Albany
Albany Medical Center Hospital
Veterans Administration Medical Center

Binghamton
Our Lady of Lourdes Memorial Hospital
United Health Services

Bronx
Bronx–Lebanon Hospital Center
Our Lady of Mercy Medical Center
Veterans Administration Medical Center

Bronxville
Lawrence Hospital

Brooklyn
Brookdale Hospital Medical Center
Brooklyn Hospital
Caledonian Hospital
Coney Island Hospital
Interfaith Medical Center
Kings County Hospital Center
Long Island College Hospital
Lutheran Medical Center
Maimonides Medical Center
Methodist Hospital
University Hospital of Brooklyn
Wyckoff Heights Hospital

Buffalo
Roswell Park Memorial Institute
Veterans Administration Medical Center

Cooperstown
Mary Imogene Bassett Hospital

East Meadow
Nassau County Medical Center

Elmhurst
City Hospital Center at Elmhurst
St. Johns Queens Hospital Division of CMC

Elmira
Arnot–Ogden Memorial Hospital
St. Joseph's Hospital

Flushing
Booth Memorial Medical Center
Flushing Hospital & Medical Center

Forest Hills
La Guardia Hospital

Glen Cove
Community Hospital at Glen Cove

Ithaca
Tompkins Community Hospital

Jamaica
Jamaica Hospital
Mary Immaculate Hospital Division of CMC
Queens Hospital Center

Jamestown
Woman's Christian Association Hospital

Manhasset
North Shore University Hospital

Mineola
Winthrop–University Hospital

Mount Kisco
Northern Westchester Hospital Center

Mount Vernon
Mount Vernon Hospital

New Hyde Park
Long Island Jewish Medical Center

New Rochelle
New Rochelle Hospital Medical Center

New York
Bellevue Hospital Center
Beth Israel Medical Center
Cabrini Medical Center
Harlem Hospital Center
Manhattan EE&T Hospital
Memorial Hospital for Cancer
Montefiore Medical Center/Moses Division
New York Infirmary/Beekman Downtown Hospital
New York University Medical Center
Presbyterian Hospital in New York City
St. Vincent's Hospital & Medical Center
Veterans Administration Medical Center

Oceanside
South Nassau Communities Hospital

Patchogue
Brookhaven Memorial Hospital Medical Center

Appendix 2

NEW YORK (*Cont.*)

Plainview
  Central General Hospital
Port Jefferson
  John T. Mather Memorial Hospital
  St. Charles Hospital
Port Jervis
  Mercy Community Hospital
Poughkeepsie
  Vassar Brothers Hospital
Rochester
  Genesee Hospital
  Highland Hospital of Rochester
  Park Ridge Hospital
  Rochester General Hospital
  Rochester St. Mary's Hospital
Rockville Centre
  Mercy Hospital
Schenectady
  Ellis Hospital
Staten Island
  Bayley Seton Hospital
  St. Vincent's Medical Center
  Staten Island Hospital
Stony Brook
  University Hospital, SUNY
Suffern
  Good Samaritan Hospital
Syracuse
  St. Joseph's Hospital Health Center
  SUNY Health Science Center
Troy
  Samaritan Hospital
Valhalla
  Westchester County Medical Center
Valley Stream
  Franklin General Hospital
Walton
  Delaware Valley Hospital

NORTH CAROLINA

Asheville
  Memorial Mission Hospital
Camp Lejeune
  Naval Hospital
Chapel Hill
  North Carolina Memorial Hospital
Durham
  Duke University Hospital
Shelby
  Cleveland Memorial Hospital

Valdese
  Valdese General Hospital
Winston-Salem
  North Carolina Baptist Hospital

NORTH DAKOTA

Bismark
  Medcenter One
  St. Alexius Medical Center
Fargo
  Dakota Hospital/Dakota Clinic
  St. John's Hospital
  St. Luke's Hospitals
  Veterans Administration Center
Grand Forks
  United Hospital
Mandan
  Mandan Hospital
Minot
  St. Joseph's Hospital
Rugby
  Good Samaritan Hospital
    Association
Williston
  Mercy Medical Center & Hospital

OHIO

Akron
  Akron City Hospital
  Akron General Medical Center
  St. Thomas Hospital Medical
    Center
Barberton
  Barberton Citizens Hospital
Canton
  Aultman Hospital
  Timken Mercy Medical Center
Chardon
  Geauga Community Hospital
Cincinnati
  Bethesda Oak Hospital
  Children's Hospital Medical Center
  Christ Hospital
  Good Samaritan Hospital
  Jewish Hospital of Cincinnati
  St. Francis–St. George Hospital
  University of Cincinnati Hospital
Cleveland
  Cleveland Clinic Hospital
  Cleveland Metropolitan General
    Hospital

Deaconess Hospital of Cleveland
Huron Road Hospital
Lutheran Medical Center
Mount Sinai Medical Center
St. Alexis Hospital
St. Vincent Charity Hospital
University Hospitals of Cleveland
Columbus
Children's Hospital
Grant Medical Center
Mount Carmel Health
Ohio State University Hospitals
Riverside Methodist Hospitals
St. Anthony Medical Center
Dayton
Good Samaritan Hospital & Health
Center
Miami Valley Hospital
St. Elizabeth Medical Center
Dover
Union Hospital
Elyria
Elyria Memorial Hospital
Gallipolis
Holzer Medical Center
Kettering
Kettering Medical Center
Lima
St. Rita's Medical Center
Lorain
St. Joseph Hospital & Health
Center
Marion
Marion General Hospital
Mayfield Heights
Hillcrest Hospital
Medina
Medina Community Hospital
Middleburg Heights
Southwest Community Health
System & Hospital
Oregon
St. Charles Hospital
Parma
Parma Community General
Hospital
Ravenna
Robinson Memorial Hospital
Sandusky
Firelands Community Hospital
Providence Hospital

Springfield
Community Hospital of Springfield
Mercy Medical Center
Steubenville
Ohio Valley Hospital
Sylvania
Flower Memorial Hospital
Toledo
Medical College of Ohio Hospital
Riverside Hospital
St. Vincent Medical Center
Toledo Hospital
Urbana
Mercy Memorial Hospital
Warren
Trumbull Memorial Hospital
Wright-Patterson Air Force Base
U.S. Air Force Medical Center
Xenia
Greene Memorial Hospital
Youngstown
St. Elizabeth Hospital Medical
Center
Western Reserve Care Systems
Zanesville
Bethesda Hospital
Good Samaritan Medical Center

OKLAHOMA
Ada
Valley View Regional Hospital
Bartlesville
Jane Phillips Episcopal–Memorial
Medical Center
Chickasha
Grady Memorial Hospital
Lawton
AMI Southwestern Medical Center
Muskogee
Muskogee Regional Medical
Center
Oklahoma City
Baptist Medical Center of
Oklahoma
Mercy Health Center
Oklahoma Children's Memorial
Hospital
Oklahoma Memorial Hospital
Presbyterian Hospital
South Community Hospital
St. Anthony Hospital

169

OKLAHOMA (*Cont.*)
Shattuck
Newman Memorial Hospital
Shawnee
Shawnee Medical Center Hospital
Tulsa
Hillcrest Medical Center
St. Francis Hospital
St. John Medical Center

OREGON
Albany
Albany General Hospital
Bend
St. Charles Medical Center
Clackamas
Kaiser Foundation Hospitals—
NW Region
Corvallis
Good Samaritan Hospital
Eugene
Sacred Heart General Hospital
Grants Pass
Josephine Memorial Hospital
Klamath Falls
Merle West Medical Center
Medford
Providence Hospital
Rogue Valley Memorial Hospital
Oregon City
Willamette Falls Hospital
Pendleton
St. Anthony Hospital
Portland
Emanuel Hospital & Health Center
Good Samaritan Hospital &
Medical Center
Oregon Health Sciences University
Hospital
Portland Adventist Medical Center
Providence Medical Center
St. Vincent Hospital & Medical
Center
Veterans Administration Medical
Center
Roseburg
Douglas Community Hospital
Mercy Medical Center
Salem
Salem Hospital

Tualatin
Meridian Park Hospital

PENNSYLVANIA
Allentown
Allentown Hospital
Lehigh Valley Hospital Center
Sacred Heart Hospital
Altoona
Altoona Hospital
Mercy Hospital
Beaver
The Medical Center
Bethlehem
St. Luke's Hospital
Bryn Mawr
Bryn Mawr Hospital
Chester
Crozer-Chester Medical Center
Danville
Geisinger Medical Center
Drexel Hill
Delaware County Memorial
Hospital
Easton
Easton Hospital
Erie
Hamot Medical Center
Franklin
Franklin Regional Medical Center
Greensburg
Westmoreland Hospital
Greenville Regional Hospital
Hershey
Pennsylvania State University
Hospital
Johnstown
Conemaugh Valley Memorial
Hospital
Lancaster
Lancaster General Hospital
St. Joseph Hospital
Lansdale
North Penn Hospital
Latrobe
Latrobe Area Hospital
Lewistown
Lewistown Hospital
Natrona Heights
Allegheny Valley Hospital

New Castle
  Jameson Memorial Hospital
Norristown
  Montgomery Hospital
  Sacred Heart Hospital
Paoli
  Paoli Memorial Hospital
Philadelphia
  AEMC Mount Sinai–Daroff Division
  AEMC North Division
  American Oncologic Hospital
  Childrens Hospital of Philadelphia
  Episcopal Hospital
  Graduate Hospital
  Hahnemann University Hospital
  Hospital of the Medical College of
    Pennsylvania
  Jeanes Hospital
  Mercy Catholic Medical Center
  Northeastern Hospital of
    Philadelphia
  Pennsylvania Hospital
  Temple University Hospital
  Thomas Jefferson University
    Hospital
Pittsburgh
  Allegheny General Hospital
  Children's Hospital of Pittsburgh
  Eye and Ear Hospital of Pittsburgh
  Magee–Women's Hospital
  Mercy Hospital of Pittsburgh
  Presbyterian–University Hospital
  St. Francis Medical Center
Pottstown
  Pottstown Memorial Medical
    Center
Pottsville
  Pottsville Hospital & Warne Clinic
Quakertown
  Quakertown Community Hospital
Reading
  Community General Hospital
  Reading Hospital & Medical
    Center
  St. Joseph Hospital
Sayre
  Robert Packer Hospital
Scranton
  Mercy Hospital of Scranton
  Moses Taylor Hospital

Sellersville
  Grand View Hospital
State College
  Centre Community Hospital
Tunkhannock
  Tyler Memorial Hospital
West Chester
  Chester County Hospital
Wilkes-Barre
  Veterans Administration Medical
    Center
Williamsport
  Divine Providence Hospital
  Williamsport Hospital & Medical
    Center
York
  York Hospital

PUERTO RICO
Mayaguez
  Mayaguez Medical Center
Ponce
  Hospital de Damas
  Hospital Onco Andres Grillasca
San German
  Hospital de la Concepcion
San Juan
  I. Gonzalez Martinez Onco
    Hospital
  University Hospital
  Veterans Administration Medical
    Center

RHODE ISLAND
Newport
  Naval Hospital
Providence
  Rhode Island Hospital
  Roger Williams General
    Hospital
Warwick
  Kent County Memorial Hospital

SOUTH CAROLINA
Aiken
  HCA Aiken Regional Medical
    Center
Anderson
  Anderson Memorial Hospital

171

SOUTH CAROLINA (*Cont.*)

Charleston
MUSC Medical Center of Medical
   University of South Carolina
Columbia
Baptist Medical Center
Richland Memorial Hospital
Wm. Jennings Bryan Dorn Veteran
   Hospital
Florence
McLeod Regional Medical Center
Fort Jackson
Moncrief Army Community
   Hospital
Greenville
Greenville Hospital System
Greenwood
Self Memorial Hospital
Orangeburg
Orangeburg–Calhoun Regional
   Hospital
Spartanburg
Spartanburg Medical Center

SOUTH DAKOTA

Aberdeen
St. Luke's Hospital
Rapid City
Rapid City Regional Hospital
Sioux Falls
McKennan Hospital
Sioux Valley Hospital
Watertown
Prairie Lakes Hospital East
Prairie Lakes Hospital West
Yankton
Sacred Heart Hospital

TENNESSEE

Bristol
Bristol Memorial Hospital
Chattanooga
Erlanger Medical Center
Johnson City
Johnson City Medical Center
   Hospital
Kingsport
Holston Valley Hospital & Medical
   Center

Knoxville
East Tennessee Baptist Hospital
Fort Sanders Regional Medical
   Center
University of Tennessee Memorial
   Hospital
Memphis
Baptist Memorial Hospital
Methodist Hospital—Central Unit
Regional Medical Center at
   Memphis
St. Francis Hospital
St. Jude Childrens Research
   Hospital
University of Tennessee Medical
   Center
Millington
Naval Hospital
Mountain Home
Veterans Administration Medical
   Center
Nashville
George W. Hubbard Hospital
Metropolitan Nashville General
   Hospital
Vanderbilt University Hospital

TEXAS

Amarillo
High Plains Baptist Hospital
Northwest Texas Hospital
St. Anthony's Hospital
Veterans Administration Medical
   Center
Austin
Holy Cross Hospital
Beaumont
St. Elizabeth Hospital
Big Spring
Veterans Administration Medical
   Center
Carswell Air Force Base
U.S. Air Force Regional Hospital
Corpus Christi
Memorial Medical Center
Spohn Hospital
Dallas
Baylor University Medical Center
Methodist Medical Center
Parkland Memorial Hospital

Presbyterian Hospital
St. Paul Medical Center

El Paso
Providence Memorial Hospital
R. E. Thomason General Hospital
William Beaumont Army Medical
Center

Fort Sam Houston
Brooke Army Medical Center

Galveston
University of Texas Medical Branch
Hospital

Harlingen
Valley Baptist Medical Center

Hereford
Deaf Smith General Hospital

Houston
AMI Park Plaza Hospital
Ben Taub General Hospital
Methodist Hospital
St. Joseph Hospital
University of Texas M. D. Anderson
Hospital

Lackland Air Force Base
Wilford Hall U.S. Air Force Medical
Center

Lubbock
Highland Hospital
Lubbock General Hospital
Methodist Hospital

McAllen
McAllen Medical Center

Midland
Midland Memorial Hospital

Odessa
Medical Center Hospital

Pasadena
HCA Pasadena Bayshore Medical
Center

Plainview
Central Plains Regional Hospital

San Angelo
Angelo Community Hospital

San Antonio
Audie L. Murphy Memorial Veterans
Hospital
Medical Center Hospital
Santa Rosa Medical Center
Southwest Texas Methodist
Hospital

Temple
King's Daughters Hospital
Olin E. Teague Veterans' Center
Scott and White Memorial Hospital

Waco
Hillcrest Baptist Medical Center
Providence Hospital

Wharton
Gulf Coast Medical Center

UTAH

Murray
Cottonwood Hospital Medical
Center

Salt Lake City
Holy Cross Hospital
LDS Hospital
St. Mark's Hospital
University of Utah Hospital Health
Science Center
Veterans Administration Medical
Center

West Valley City
Pioneer Valley Hospital

VERMONT

Bennington
Southwestern Vermont Medical
Center

Burlington
Medical Center Hospital of
Vermont

Randolph
Gifford Memorial Hospital

Rutland
Rutland Regional Medical Center

VIRGINIA

Alexandria
Alexandria Hospital

Arlington
Arlington Hospital
HCA Northern Virginia Hospital

Big Stone Gap
Lonesome Pine Hospital

Charlottesville
University of Virginia Hospital

Chesapeake
Chesapeake General Hospital

VIRGINIA (*Cont.*)

Danville
Memorial Hospital

Fairfax
Fair Oaks Hospital

Falls Church
Fairfax Hospital

Fredericksburg
Mary Washington Hospital

Hampton
Veterans Administration Medical Center

Harrisonburg
Rockingham Memorial Hospital

Leesburg
Loudoun Memorial Hospital

Lynchburg
Lynchburg General Hospital
Virginia Baptist Hospital

Manassas
Prince William Hospital

Martinsville
Memorial Hospital of Martinsville

Newport News
Riverside Hospital

Norfolk
DePaul Hospital
Sentara Regional Hospital

Portsmouth
Maryview Hospital
Naval Hospital
Portsmouth General Hospital

Richmond
Medical College of Virginia Hospitals
Richmond Memorial Hospital
St. Mary's Hospital

Roanoke
Community Hospital of Roanoke Valley
Roanoke Memorial Hospitals

Salem
Lewis-Gale Hospital
Veterans Administration Medical Center

Suffolk
Louise Obici Memorial Hospital

Virginia Beach
Virginia Beach General Hospital

Winchester
Winchester Medical Center

WASHINGTON

Aberdeen
Grays Harbor Community Hospital
St. Joseph Hospital

Anacortes
Island Hospital

Auburn
Auburn General Hospital

Bellevue
Overlake Hospital Medical Center

Bellingham
St. Joseph Hospital
St. Luke's General Hospital

Bremerton
Harrison Memorial Hospital
Naval Hospital

Coupeville
Whidbey General Hospital

Edmonds
Stevens Memorial Hospital

Everett
General Hospital of Everett
Providence Hospital

Kennewick
Kennewick General Hospital

Kirkland
Evergreen Hospital Medical Center

Longview
St. John's Medical Center

Mount Vernon
Skagit Valley Hospital & Health Center

Olympia
St. Peter Hospital

Pasco
Our Lady of Lourdes Health Center

Puyallup
Good Samaritan Community Healthcare

Seattle
Children's Orthopedic Hospital
Group Health Cooperative Central Hospital
Highline Community Hospital
Pacific Medical Center
Providence Medical Center
Swedish Hospital Medical Center
Virginia Mason Hospital

Sedro Woolley
United General Hospital

Spokane
  Deaconess Medical Center—
    Spokane
  Holy Family Hospital
  Sacred Heart Medical Center
Tacoma
  Madigan Army Medical Center
  St. Joseph Hospital & Health Care
    Center
  Tacoma General Hospital
Vancouver
  Southwest Washington Hospitals
Walla Walla
  St. Mary Medical Center
  Walla Walla General Hospital
Wenatchee
  Wenatchee Valley Clinic
Yakima
  St. Elizabeth Medical Center
  Yakima Valley Memorial Hospital

WEST VIRGINIA
Charleston
  Charleston Area Medical Center
Clarksburg
  Louis A. Johnson Veterans
    Administraion Medical Center
Huntington
  St. Mary's Hospital
  Veterans Administration Medical
    Center
Morgantown
  West Virginia University Hospital
Parkersburg
  Camden–Clark Memorial Hospital
Wheeling
  Ohio Valley Medical Center
  Wheeling Hospital

WISCONSIN
Appleton
  Appleton Medical Center
  St. Elizabeth Hospital

Cudahy
  Trinity Memorial Hospital
Eau Claire
  Luther Hospital
  Sacred Heart Hospital
Fond du Lac
  St. Agnes Hospital
Green Bay
  St. Vincent Hospital
Janesville
  Mercy Hospital of Janesville
La Crosse
  Lutheran Hospital—La Crosse
  St. Francis Medical Center
Madison
  Meriter Hospital
Marshfield
  Marshfield Clinic/St. Joseph's
Milwaukee
  Clement J. Zablocki Medical Center
  Columbia Hospital
  Good Samaritan Medical Center
  Milwaukee County Medical
    Complex
  Mount Sinai Medical Center
  St. Joseph's Hospital
  St. Luke's Hospital
  St. Michael Hospital
Monroe
  St. Clare Hospital of Monroe
Oshkosh
  Mercy Medical Center
Waukesha
  Waukesha Memorial Hospital
Wausau
  Wausau Hospital Center
West Allis
  West Allis Memorial Hospital

WYOMING
Cheyenne
  De Paul Hospital
  Memorial Hospital of Laramie
    County

∼ About the Author ∼

Dr. John F. Potter founded and was the first director of the Vincent T. Lombardi Cancer Research Center of Georgetown University in Washington, D.C. He is also Professor of Surgery at Georgetown.

He is the Chairman of the Board and immediate past president of the Association of American Cancer Institutes. Dr. Potter is a member of the Commission on Cancer of the American College of Surgeons. A member also of the Society of Surgical Oncology, he belongs to Alpha Omega Alpha, the national medical honorary fraternity and has been awarded the title of Professor Honorario from the Universidad Peruana Cayetano Heredia in Lima, Peru.

His numerous writings on cancer have appeared in major scientific publications, including *Cancer, The Annals of Surgery, Cancer Research,* the *New England Journal of Medicine* and the *Journal of the National Cancer Institute.*

A graduate of Holy Cross College and the Georgetown School of Medicine, Dr. Potter has served in the United States Navy and is a Knight of Malta. He is married to the former Tanya A. Kristof. They have three children; Tanya, Muffie and John.